$24⁰⁰

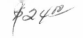

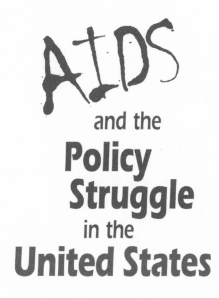

AIDS
and the
Policy
Struggle
in the
United States

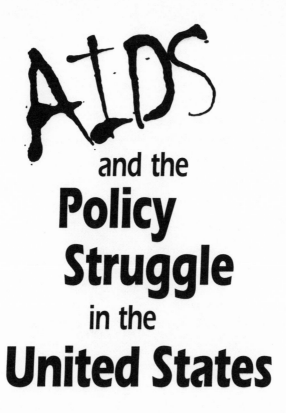

AIDS

and the
Policy
Struggle
in the
United States

Patricia D. Siplon

Georgetown University Press
Washington, D.C.

Georgetown University Press, Washington, D.C.

© 2002 by Georgetown University Press. All rights reserved.

Printed in the United States of America.

10 9 8 7 6 5 4 3 2 1   2002

This volume is printed on acid-free offset book paper.

Library of Congress Cataloging-in-Publication Data

Siplon, Patricia.

  AIDS and the policy struggle in the United States / Patricia D. Siplon.

    p.cm.

Includes bibliographical references and index.

  ISBN 0-87840-378-7 (pbk. : alk. paper) — ISBN 0-87840-377-9 (cl. :
alk. paper)

 1.   Aids (Disease)—Government policy—United States. I. Title.

  RA643.83 .S575 2002

  362.1'969793—dc21

                                            2002190217

To my husband Todd

Contents

Acknowledgments

Much of the original motivation for writing this book came from two sources. First was the desire to offer my students an accessible exploration of many of the important AIDS policy issue areas in the United States. A second motivation stemmed from a personal belief that AIDS activism, though widely written about in various disciplines and subfields, had been largely written out of our discussion of AIDS as a policy issue. Yet although this book was meant to have some benefit to students and activists (and I hope it does), I find that it is I who has benefited disproportionately from both groups in the writing of this book.

As a first-time book author, I have discovered the truth in the adages about the magnitude of emotional and intellectual debt a writer incurs. I would like to thank my students for the many great comments and questions that influenced this text. I owe a particular note of gratitude to the members of my fall 2000 and 2001 senior seminars for their careful reading and critique of drafts of many of the chapters here. I also owe a special note of thanks to Clifford Lubitz for his generous research assistance and equally valuable personal insights into the impact of HIV/AIDS as it is being experienced in sub-Saharan Africa.

I also am grateful for the support I received from many quarters within Saint Michael's College during the writing of this book. I would like to thank the Faculty Development Committee, the Center for Social Science Research, and the Office of Provost Janet Sheeran for financial support for conducting interviews and research. I am grateful to support from my departmental colleagues, particularly Kristin Novotny, whose constant friendship, superior word processing skills, and excellent imagination prevailed over a multitude of snags during the writing process. In addition, I would like to thank Sue Kuntz, Sharon Lamb, and Susan Ouellette for their careful reading of several chapters within the book. Although they work at other institutions, I also would like to thank my colleagues Paul Harris, Lilly Goren, and Lori Brainard for their support and for cheerfully putting up with lapsed deadlines and unanswered e-mails during times when I was feeling overwhelmed.

Many activists and policy advocates have taken time out of their lives to be interviewed and to provide background and information on a vast array of issues. Within the hemophilia community I am particularly indebted to Dave Cavanaugh, Michael Davon, Corey Dubin, Tom Fahey, April Klein, Dana Kuhn, Greg Malia, and Todd Smith, all of whom agreed to interviews or furnished valuable information. My knowledge of the Ryan White Act was greatly expanded through interviews with Wayne Turner of ACT UP/Washington, D.C., and Roland Foster, who works on the U.S. House of Representatives Subcommittee on Criminal Justice, Drug Policy and Human Resources. Although they are of very different ideological turns, both men were exceptionally helpful in interviews and in sharing information. Roland also provided me with extensive information about HIV testing among infants.

I owe the largest debt of all to ACT UP/New York, ACT UP/Philadelphia, and Health GAP. The people in these organizations have not only produced volumes of valuable information on the issues of treatment access and affordability in the United States and developing countries, they also are largely responsible for bringing greater awareness of these issues into the national policy arena. There are too many names to list here, but I am grateful to the many individuals within these groups who have produced documentation, explanations, and answers to volumes of questions. Their energy is not only enormous, it is contagious, and members of these groups have inspired a great many other individuals and organizations to join the AIDS policy struggle. I hope that some of the expertise, passion, and creativity of these groups will show through in the pages that follow.

On a personal level, I also would like to thank a few people for their guidance and forbearance. I am grateful to Tom Baldino and Deborah Stone for their many kindnesses as mentors. I would like to thank John Tierney for his efforts on my behalf, as well as on behalf of this book. I also would like to extend my appreciation to the folks at Georgetown University Press, especially Gail Grella, as well as a very helpful anonymous reviewer.

Finally, I would like to thank my family, particularly three people. My sister Katrinka has always been an unflagging supporter of my original choice to study AIDS as a political scientist and of just about every word I've written since. My father Donald, despite his strong disagreements with many of my conclusions, instilled in me my interest in public health and health policy and taught me by example the value of taking part in the policy process. My husband, Todd Watkins, served as a sounding board for ideas, edited much of the text in earlier forms, and reined in my prose before I went off on too many tangents. He also exemplified the very meaning of support by spending the first Valentine's Day of our married life not with wine and roses but sitting in my office with me, proofing pages to make a deadline. I am lucky to have had such an unstinting source of support in my life, and to him I gratefully dedicate this book.

Abbreviations

AABB	American Association of Blood Banks
ABRA	American Blood Resource Association
ACBSA	Advisory Committee on Blood Safety and Availability
ACES	AIDS Community Educators
ACLU	American Civil Liberties Union
ACTG 076	AIDS Clinical Trial Group Protocol 076
ACT UP	AIDS Coalition to Unleash Power
ADAP	AIDS Drug Assistance Program
ADAPT	Association for Drug Abuse Prevention and Treatment
AFLA	Adolescent Family Life Act
AGOA	African Growth and Opportunities Act
AHF	antihemophilia factor
AIDS	acquired immunodeficiency syndrome
AMA	American Medical Association
AmFAR	American Foundation for AIDS Research
ANRC	American National Red Cross
APHA	American Public Health Association
ARC	AIDS Resource Center
AZT	azidothymidine
BNC	Binational Commission
BPAC	Blood Products Advisory Committee
CAEAR	Cities Advocating Emergency AIDS Relief
CARE	Comprehensive AIDS Resource Emergency
CCBC	Council of Community Blood Centers
CBER	Center for Biologics Evaluation and Research
CDC	Centers for Disease Control and Prevention
COTT	Committee of Ten Thousand
DECA	Distributive Education Clubs of America
EMA	eligible metropolitan area
FDA	Food and Drug Administration
GAA	Global AIDS Alliance
GAO	General Accounting Office
GAP	Global Access Project
GDP	gross domestic product
GMHC	Gay Men's Health Crisis
GRID	gay-related immune deficiency
GTAC	Global Treatment Action Campaign

HAART	highly active antiretroviral therapy
HCFA	Health Care Financing Administration
HELP	Senate/Committee Health, Education, Labor, and Pension
H/HIV	Hemophilia/HIV
HHS	Department of Health and Human Services
HHSPC	HIV Health Services Planning Council
HIV	human immunodeficiency virus
HOPE	Human Rights, Opportunity, Partnership and Empowerment Act
HRSA	Health Resources and Services Administration
HTC	hemophilia treatment center
HTLV	human T-cell leukemia virus
IND	investigational new drug
IOM	Institute of Medicine
KSOI	Kaposi's sarcoma—opportunistic infection
LAV	lymphadenopathy-associated virus
LIFE	Leadership in Fighting an Epidemic
MANN	Man's Advocacy Network of NHF
MASAC	Medical and Scientific Advisory Committee
MED4ALL	Global Right to Vital Medicines—Medicine for All
MSF	*Medecins San Frontieres*
NAPWA	National Association of People With Aids
NAVTA	National Association for Victims of Transfusion-Acquired AIDS
NCI	National Cancer Institute
NDA	new drug application
NEP	needle-exchange program
NHF	National Hemophilia Foundation
NHLBI	National Heart, Lung and Blood Institute
NIAID	National Institute for Allergies and Infectious Diseases
NIDA	National Institute on Drug Abuse
NIH	National Institutes of Health
NORA	National Organizations Responding to AIDS
NOW	National Organization for Women
NSC	National Security Council
OVP	Office of the Vice President
PCP	*Pneumocystis carinii* pneumonia
PhRMA	Pharmaceutical Research and Manufacturers of America
PUC	Plasma Users Coalition
PWA	people with AIDS
SAC	Special Assistance Council
SAG	Government of South Africa
SDI	strategic (or structured) drug interruption
SPNS	Special Projects of National Significance

STD	sexually transmitted disease
STI	strategic treatment interruption
TAC	Treatment Action Campaign
TANF	Temporary Assistance to Needy Families
TRIPS	Trade Related Aspects of Intellectual Property
UCSF	University of California–San Francisco
UNAIDS	Joint United Nations Programme on HIV/AIDS
UNGASS	United Nations General Assembly Special Session
USAID	U.S. Agency for International Development
USPTO	U.S. Patent and Trademark Office
USTR	United States Trade Representative
USUHS	Uniformed Services University of Health Sciences
WHO	World Health Organization
WTO	World Trade Organization

CHAPTER 1

The Nature of the Policy Process

The policymaking process, by its very nature, is controversial. In fact, all policy is the product of struggles between groups. The term *policy*, in its simplest conception, refers to nothing more than a decision or set of decisions about how to deal with an issue or a problem. Especially when we are discussing governments and politics, we often use the term *policy* when we really mean *public policy*, which addresses the realm of decisions made by the government as opposed to private citizens and groups. Because acquired immunodeficiency syndrome (AIDS) is a communicable disease and because prevention and treatment of communicable diseases have a history of being defined at least partially as the responsibility of the government, most of the policies surrounding AIDS in the United States are, in fact, public policies. Decisions about government-funded AIDS research (what questions to ask, whom to pay to ask them), decisions about foreign assistance for countries with heavily affected populations (whether to give them money, what strings we might attach to the money we give), and decisions about government services for those infected and affected by AIDS and the human immunodeficiency virus (HIV) (what sorts of government services they need most and who should administer these services) are examples of AIDS public policies in the United States.

There also are many important private policies that heavily affect people with AIDS and HIV, however. These policies include decisions by private pharmaceutical companies about how much to charge for AIDS medications and to whom to make them available; decisions by private physicians about how to manage their relationships with patients; and decisions by philanthropic organizations about whether to fund public education materials containing sexually explicit information about HIV transmission. Still other decisions occupy a gray area because they involve decision makers from the private and public (government) realms. Because so many private and public policy decisions are intertwined, in this book I examine policy areas that encompass more than the public policy domain that is the primary area of interest to students of U.S. politics and policy.

Many books about policy begin with a model of policymaking that is based on rational decision making. According to such models, the government—or whoever is in charge of making the all-important policy decisions—goes through a set of rational steps to achieve policy solutions. Such steps might include identifying the problem, identifying alternative solutions to the problem, weighing each solution, and selecting the solution with the least cost and the most benefits.[1] Although this model is common, it is not the one I propose for viewing the HIV/AIDS policy process. Instead, I suggest that we think about the development of policies regarding HIV and AIDS as analogous to a chaotic version of the Olympic Games. Various matches are being held simultaneously, and new players may be called into the games when coaches see that their side appears to be losing or gaining ground. Others, like the sprinter who foregoes the 400-meter race to save her strength for a 200-meter race, may pull out of a policy contest to concentrate their resources on a different one. Some matches have many spectators cheering from the sidelines; others are being conducted in front of relatively few. Members of the government, who were originally called in as unbiased judges and referees, may find themselves taking sides. Indeed, as in the Olympics themselves, even the venue where the struggles will take place may be a highly contested issue. Like the cities that compete to host the games, policy groups often compete to have decision making occur in their arena, on their terms. Policy combatants may find that what seems to be a victory or solution carries within it the seeds of a defeat or new problem, like the valiant athlete who decides to carry on with an injury, only to be sidelined when the condition worsens. And sometimes, when a match is over, the disgruntled losers demand a rematch, arguing that the results of the original were unfair or simply undesirable.

This metaphor for policymaking has important implications:

- Many policy struggles over a given issue are going on at once. Sometimes the actors have to play them out simultaneously and make strategic decisions on where to put their resources.
- The results of policy decisions are not "objective." They are the result of contests between people and groups with very different perspectives, whose relative strengths in the policy process can wax and wane over time.
- The government, the ultimate decision-making body for most public policy, also is not "objective." Actors who are engaged in policymaking contests heavily influence the government in many ways.
- The results of a policy decision are not final, strictly speaking. In policy as in sports, winners may be satisfied with the outcome, but losers seldom are. The side that perceives itself as losing will regroup and look for another opportunity or time to reopen the issue. And, as in sports, winners also become targets to beat in later contests.
- In many cases, "solutions" only create new problems.
- Finally, the actors themselves are not static. Some of them will drop out of the struggle, some may even change sides, and new actors (perhaps even the readers of a book such as this) will emerge to take their places.

Whenever decisions are made (regardless of whether the decision makers are private, governmental, or some combination of both), there are winners and losers. In a world in which there is never enough time, money, talent, or energy, a decision to expend some of these resources in a given direction will necessarily leave someone—or, more often, some group—asking why these resources weren't spent differently. If the group asking this question is angry, frightened, or otherwise motivated enough, it may even get organized and demand a reconsideration of the decision. And the decision may or may not move in a new direction. This is the nature of the policy struggle.

To more completely understand the general nature of the policy process, we must always keep in mind three key elements that will strongly affect the direction in which different policies will move: the role of organization, the role of values, and the problem of changing distributions and inflicting costs on affected groups and society in general. Although the interplay of these elements, as well as examples of each, appear often throughout the book, each merits a few words of introduction.

The issue of organization is fundamental for the study of policy, and a great many scholars have fashioned theories about how the organization of groups affects the policy outputs of governments (as well as the policy outputs of nongovernmental actors). For example, the train of thought known as pluralism suggests that when groups of people have a collective need or grievance, they will choose to organize and take their requests to government.[2] Other scholars have suggested that this idea is over optimistic and that there are barriers that must be overcome if people are to organize collectively. One famous barrier is the "free rider problem" that occurs when individuals realize that if others donate their time and organizational energies, they can enjoy the benefits without joining and doing the work (thereby "free riding").[3] A more recent argument has surfaced that a barrier to current organizing efforts in the United States derives from our low reserves of "social capital"—the social networks that bind us together and, according to this argument, have diminished drastically over the past twenty-five years.[4] In this book I examine a wide spectrum of groups that have overcome these obstacles (as well as a few cases in which organization hasn't happened, though it might have been a great benefit to would-be group members).

Importantly, when we examine the organizing of various actors we must look at more than the financial resources they have at their disposal (although that factor certainly plays a major role in many conflicts). We also must examine other, less tangible, resources, such as members' commitment to one another and to the group's objectives and members' willingness to engage in action outside of the conventional (what scholars who study social movements often refer to as engaging in "contentious politics").

Such considerations also bring us into exploration of the second key idea: the role of values. All policy decisions in some way reflect the values of the society (or a significant subset of the society) in which they are produced. Much of our current AIDS policy, however, represents the product of particularly value-laden struggles. The values of freedom, security, tolerance, equity, and democracy probably are all valued by Americans in the abstract. We run into problems, however, when we move into the realm of concrete policy choices. One problem arises when different individuals and groups have differing interpretations of what, exactly, is meant when a given value is invoked. A second conflict occurs because of the unfortunate truism that we can't have everything at once once. Thus, although we all may value many ideals simultaneously, when we make policy choices we must choose some values over others.

Finally, as with all policy areas, the creation and evolution of AIDS policy entails the distribution and redistribution of resources and the imposition of costs. Obviously, all groups have a desire to secure resources (usually money, but sometimes decision-making authority, attention, and other social goods) and avoid costs.

All groups also believe that they have logical arguments for why they are most deserving of these resources and of avoiding having the costs inflicted upon them. Usually these resources and costs are meted out by government bodies. Thus, these bodies have the unpopular job of saying "yes" to some groups and "no" to others.

Although at first glance there might seem to be obvious ways to make these decisions (for example, give resources to the people who need them most or to the groups with the most people), the reality is very different. As I seek to demonstrate in this book, all kinds of other "nonobjective" characteristics go into decision making. Which groups are already getting resources? How long have groups managed to avoid having costs inflicted on them? Who is paying attention when decisions are being made? The answers to these types of questions have important effects on how resources and costs will be distributed.

Special Features of the AIDS Policy Process

This country's AIDS policies (that is, the collection of decisions made in the United States about how to prevent the spread of HIV infection and treat people who have become infected) have been the product of a particularly contentious policy struggle. There are many reasons that the struggles around AIDS policy stand out as particularly hard-fought and newsworthy. First, AIDS was first recognized in the United States among people who belonged to groups that tended to have either little political power or negative associations in the minds of "mainstream" Americans: sexually active gay men, intravenous drug users, Haitian immigrants, and people with hemophilia. When some of these groups chose to develop and flex their political muscles, it made news—and often forced a rethinking of decisions about the ways in which the newly emerging disease should be handled.

Another reason that AIDS has been such a contentious and high-profile area of policy struggle is that the stakes are very high. Even before AIDS had a name, people knew that it was a frightening, life-threatening problem. Many of the struggles over the development of AIDS policy have been literally life-and-death contests. Deciding either to ignore or pour money into researching the mysterious new condition; selecting which manifestations of the disease to explore and later how much to charge for life-saving new medications; choosing whether to write sexually explicit pamphlets and engage in illegal needle exchanges for the sake of preventing the spread of HIV: These are just a few of the many times when those infected or affected by HIV perceived that lives would be saved or lost depending on the choices that were ultimately made.

Less dramatic, though extremely important, is the fact that lifestyles also are deeply affected by AIDS policy choices. Just as people will fight very hard to preserve their lives and those of their loved ones, so they will fight to preserve their values and the values of their communities. The particular circumstances of AIDS—the communities in which it was first discovered, the way it is transmitted, and its often fatal nature—brought communities with very different values into direct conflict with one another. Thus, members of the public health community and elements of the gay community initially engaged in bitter debate. It was hard for many public health professionals, who had always dealt with infectious diseases by finding infected individuals and trying to limit their opportunities for infecting others, to understand elements of the gay community, who sought to preserve their sexual freedom and thus fought hard to keep open bath houses and other places that facilitated sexual encounters. Similarly, religious leaders and their congregations, who had always advocated monogamous sexual relationships within marriage, found themselves unable to come to terms with members of the public health and gay communities who sought to offer explicit instructions to adults and teenagers of all sexual orientations about "safer sex." What is at issue in such policy struggles is more than the pragmatic questions of how to most expeditiously stop the transmission of a virus. The communities in these and many other AIDS-related policy struggles are seeking to validate and preserve values and ways of living.

A third reason that AIDS-related policy struggles have been so hard-fought is that they have involved change. Obviously, the process of policy making often involves change. AIDS policies have been extreme in this regard, however. The traditional approach to containing infectious disease, particularly sexually transmitted disease, has relied heavily on a combination of coercive measures and moralistic messages. Often, especially if the disease occurred mainly within marginalized groups or was believed to spread through morally suspect behavior, society blamed the victim for becoming infected or transmitting the disease to others.[5] Although the initial response to AIDS from society and the government was similar to previous responses to such disease, the reaction from the people it infected was very different. Confronted with a disease that disproportionately affected certain demographic groups, one of these groups—sexually active gay men, together with the larger gay and lesbian community—rejected the traditional approach of blame, isolation of the sick, and moralism. Instead, the gay community challenged the larger society and government to view infectious disease in a new, less judgmental way and to view societal causes, such as lack of accessible information, bigotry, and poverty, as reasons for the spread of HIV.

Similarly, approaches to policies regarding the medical treatment and management of HIV also have undergone a deep shift. Prior to the advent of AIDS, the realm of infectious disease was defined, controlled, and managed almost entirely by health professionals. AIDS activists have mounted a very effective challenge to this "ownership" of AIDS issues by medical and academic experts. By using a strategy of self-education and a philosophy of personal empowerment, they have suggested that ownership of policy issues surrounding a given disease at the very least should be shared with the people who actually are most affected by the disease. These people, they argue, by virtue of their day-to-day experience of living with HIV, as well as their enormous stake in the outcome of policy decisions, are entitled and qualified to be crucial players in AIDS policymaking circles.

Finally, AIDS activism has changed activism itself, partly as a result of some of the special circumstances of the AIDS epidemic. Many of the people infected with HIV during the early years of the epidemic, as well as those close to them, were well educated, articulate, creative, and financially well-off. Thus, they had resources of money, time, and skills that often are less available when disease occurs among, for example, people who are very poor. Similarly, especially in the urban areas of San Francisco and New York City, many early activists were well connected to larger communities that were relatively easy to mobilize to action. The successes of AIDS activists created a new model featuring direct action, self-empowerment, and self-education first for other health-based groups and ultimately even for activist groups outside the health realm.

There are many ways of looking at the AIDS epidemic, and a great many books, films, and articles have been produced that examine AIDS from scientific, personal, fictional, psychological, political, and sociological perspectives (to name a few). All of these perspectives have great value in helping us understand and deal with the problems wrought by this epidemic.[6]

In this book I examine several AIDS issues from a policy perspective. That is, I examine several issue areas to see what decisions were made by a combination of government and private actors. An important assumption of the book is that all of these decisions are the results of struggles among groups and individuals, so I also closely examine some of these struggles to see how they resulted in the policy options that ultimately were chosen.

A complete look at the AIDS epidemic in the United States is beyond the scope of this book. My plan is to examine several important policy areas, and, within each area, some of the defining struggles that occurred. In each chapter I try to pick policy examples that do three things. First, they should exemplify the larger theoretical and philosophical conflict that has occurred within a given policy area. Second, they should illustrate larger policy processes and lessons. Finally, I hope they will hold the reader's interest and demonstrate why the struggle around AIDS has made it such a divisive but also vibrant and innovative policy area.

In the rest of this chapter I outline three subjects that will help form a basis for understanding the policy issues I examine in depth in succeeding chapters. First, I introduce some of the groups that have been heavily affected by AIDS and that have in turn strongly effected AIDS policy. This introduction includes groups in and outside of government because both types have been critical to the policy process. Next I briefly outline one of the first policy struggles over AIDS: identifying its cause and outlining a research program to deal with the new disease. Finally, I very briefly overview the five policy areas (medical treatment, blood policy, transmission prevention, social service delivery, and AIDS-based foreign policy) that the book covers.

The Four H's of AIDS Politics

On March 3, 1983, after almost two years of studying an apparently new infectious disease that compromised peoples' immune systems, the Centers for Disease Control and Prevention (CDC), the U.S. government agency responsible for tracking the incidence of disease in the United States, made an official pronouncement. At that time, the agency claimed that it had identified four groups at increased risk for AIDS: homosexual men who had multiple sexual partners, intravenous heroin injectors, Haitians who had immigrated into the United States in recent years, and hemophiliacs. These groups within the AIDS 4-H Club, as they came to be satirically called, reacted to this designation in different ways.

One of the groups, Haitians, rejected the CDC classification and pushed hard to throw off any association with the new disease. The first period of protest followed the 1983 "at-risk" classification, and in 1985 the Haitian community prevailed in having the CDC remove Haitians from its list of at-risk groups. After a second intense period of protests that peaked in April 1990, the Food and Drug Administration (FDA)—the government agency responsible for the safety of the nation's blood supply—backed down and rescinded its ban on Haitian blood donation.[7] Thus, the Haitian community was able to withdraw from its association with HIV, and it became a relatively minor player in the policy struggles that occurred during the 1990s.

For different reasons, the other three groups remained strongly associated with HIV. In the hemophilia community, the association was based in very large part on the tremendously high level of infection and subsequent negative impact the community suffered beginning in the early 1980s when the infection occurred. As I discuss in some detail in chapter 3, the nature of hemophilia treatment in the 1980s, which was based on the use of products to clot blood that were derived from the unscreened plasma of thousands of paid donations, virtually guaranteed that heavy users of this factor would become HIV-infected. When this eventuality occurred, however, hemophiliacs did not immediately mobilize because they were misinformed about the prevalence of HIV infection within the community and because they were encouraged by their own advocacy groups to place confidentiality above political action. When the tide turned and mobilization did occur, the hemophilia community pursued aims that were somewhat different than the larger AIDS community's goals, such as assigning responsibility for the contamination of the blood supply and receiving compensation for the many deaths and family disruptions that resulted from that contamination. This difference of purpose sometimes has created tension between people with hemophilia and HIV and those who were infected through other means.

Like hemophiliacs, heroin users for the most part were not mobilized in the early days of the epidemic. In the United States, the obstacles to such organization were manifold. There are problems relating to the nature of drug addiction: Getting and using drugs are a higher priority for most drug addicts than other concerns, including health care and political mobilization.[8] Another obstacle to organization is the criminal nature of the activity itself and the penalties that may result from self-disclosure, which is usually a part of the process of organizing groups. Finally, there is the problem that there *is* no "drug user community," at least in the sense of a group of people with a strong sense of group identity, shared fate, and personal loyalty to one another like that enjoyed by other HIV-infected communities such as the hemophilia community.

Although drug users themselves did not organize (with some notable individual exceptions), many other actors organized to speak on their behalf. Although not all injection drug users are members of racial minority groups, of course, in many places the issue of HIV transmission facilitated by drug use was defined as a problem of minority—particularly African-American—communities. Often the African-American community found itself at odds with groups of public health professionals and AIDS advocates from within the (usually white) gay community that also had organized around the issue.

Although the African-American community's most widely publicized role in AIDS policy development has occurred around needle exchange, it has become an important policy player in other AIDS-related policy arenas as well. Though acknowledgment has been slow in coming, African-American members of the gay and lesbian community have made important contributions to the policy process from the earliest days of the epidemic, as have African-American religious institutions, although the latter were relatively less active until the mid-1990s.[9]

As for the final "H" in the club—homosexual men—mobilization was rapid and expansive. The community that came together to confront AIDS was composed of lesbians as well as gay men and HIV-negative individuals as well as people who were infected. The gay community became a major player in crafting and changing almost all of the policies that have evolved to address AIDS not only because gay men were infected with the virus (after all, infection had occurred in all of the other groups in the 4-H club) but because the gay community *decided* to take an active role in policy formation. This decision came about in part because the gay community felt that the government was not doing enough; so, through the formation of AIDS service organizations, the community sought to meet the needs of people who had AIDS. Yet the gay community also chose this course of action precisely because it did not want the government and public health professionals to do more, if "more" meant crafting policies that it feared would be discriminatory and even punitive toward members of the community.

As the epidemic has progressed, the lines between these groups have blurred, and new coalitions have sprung up that have brought individuals from different groups together. Nowhere is this more evident than with the AIDS Coalition to Unleash Power (ACT UP). This activist group has its roots within the gay community of New York City. ACT UP began in 1987 as a direct-action protest movement; chapters quickly sprang up around the country and then in other major cities around the world. ACT UP has been an important participant in many of the policies discussed in this book, including research and pricing of AIDS drug treatments, care of AIDS patients, needle exchanges, prevention and education programs, and, most recently, AIDS in the developing world. Although ACT UP initially was strongest in the two cities in the United States with the largest AIDS caseload and most active gay communities—New York City and San Francisco— that is no longer the case. The New York City chapter still exists but is smaller and garners fewer headlines than it once did, and the original members of the San Francisco chapter have left it altogether after new members who don't believe in the connection between HIV and AIDS took it over. The old members became ACT UP Golden Gate; then, in an attempt to completely dissociate with the current ACT UP San Francisco, ACT UP Golden Gate became Survive AIDS. Currently the largest and most active chapter of ACT UP in the country is ACT UP Philadelphia. ACT UP Philadelphia also is reflective of the evolution of AIDS and the groups that have become active players. Unlike the earlier large chapters in big cities, which drew their strength from the (mostly white) middle-class gay community, at least half of ACT UP Philadelphia's membership is composed of people of color, mainly drawn from low income areas of the city.

The Usual Suspects in Health Policy Struggles

AIDS policy struggles have been remarkable for their inclusion of consumers as policy players, like those introduced above, who previously had, at most, minor roles in the policy process. Government actors and health professionals, who usually play major roles in health policy issues, have hardly been relegated to the sidelines, however. They continued to have major roles in AIDS policies, though perhaps not the defining ones they had in earlier policy areas.

One of the important features of American government is that it is purposely divided in several ways. At the national level, power is divided between the Congress (which passes the laws); the executive branch, headed by the president (which carries out the laws); and the judiciary (which interprets the laws). Of these three branches, the first two have been instrumental in developing AIDS policies; the judicial branch has been less active, although it has been vital in areas such as defining what constitutes AIDS-related discrimination.

Although the president can influence public opinion, issue executive orders, and veto or sign laws, most of the AIDS-related work of the executive branch actually takes place within the Department of Health and Human Services (HHS). This cabinet department is one of fourteen within the executive branch. Other departments also play important roles, including the Department of State; one of its agencies is the U.S. Agency for International Development (USAID), through which most AIDS-related development money to other countries is funneled.

HHS, in turn, comprises other agencies that have had important AIDS-related roles. Among these is the Public Health Service, which is headed by the Surgeon General. One of the agencies within the Public Health Service that has played an extremely important ongoing role is the CDC. This agency first tracked the emerging epidemic, and it has been responsible for continuing surveillance of the epidemic, as well as prevention programs, in the United States and, increasingly, abroad.

Another important set of agencies within HHS is the National Institutes of Health (NIH). These institutes are publicly funded research entities that study major diseases. The National Institute for Allergies and Infectious Diseases (NIAID) has been particularly involved in AIDS research since the early days of the epidemic.

Still another HHS agency with a major role has been the FDA. The FDA is essentially a consumer protection agency. It makes sure that the foods we eat and the drugs we take are safe and, in the case of drugs, effective. The FDA has had multiple AIDS policy roles. It is the FDA's job to approve and license the tests we use to detect HIV. Agencies within the FDA are responsible for creating the rules that are used to maintain a safe blood supply. The FDA also has had the unenviable job of balancing safety with availability in deciding whether and when to approve the drugs that have been developed to fight HIV and its associated opportunistic infections.

Although the U.S. health care system is far more privatized than that of any other developed western nation, the U.S. government still has a very significant share of responsibility in paying for the nation's health. This is particularly true for persons who are elderly and disabled (who are supported by the nation's Medicare program) and those who are poor (who are supported by Medicaid, the joint federal/state partnership program). Because many people who become infected with HIV are poor and many more become poor or disabled because of HIV, these programs are significantly related to HIV and AIDS policies. Again, departments within HHS, particularly the Health Care Finance Administration (HCFA), carry out the work that must be done to support these programs.

Responsibilities also are shared widely on the legislative side. Congress is divided into the House of Representatives and the Senate, and each comprises numerous committees. These committees, in turn, are divided into subcommittees, which do much of the work of creating and modifying laws. The committees that deal with health issues, such as the Health Subcommittee (formerly the Health and Environment Subcommittee) of the House Committee on Energy and Commerce and the Senate Health, Education, Labor and Pension (HELP) Committee, have been particularly involved in AIDS policies. In addition to the committee structure, Congress also contains a more informal caucus system that allows members with particular interests to work together. One such caucus, the Congressional Black Caucus, has raised its collective voice on many occasions to address particular AIDS policy issues.

Like the national government, state and local governments have been very involved in AIDS policy issues. Many of the policy areas addressed in this book, including HIV testing, provision of services, AIDS education, and prevention measures are decided or partially decided at the state level. Thus, on many occasions, state legislatures, health departments, and governors, as well as city politicians—including mayors and school boards—have been important policy players.

Finally, within the private sector, medical professionals have played important roles, individually and collectively. On the individual level, health care professionals, especially doctors, have moved from a more authoritarian model of health care delivery to one that includes the patient as an equal partner in decisions regarding treatment. At the collective level, professionals—including doctors, nurses, and specialty groups such as surgeons and pediatricians—have attempted to affect policy by offering policy perspectives that are made authoritative through endorsement of entire groups, such as the American Medical Association (AMA).

Track, Identify, Treat

In retrospect, it may appear that the task of government agencies during the early years of the AIDS epidemic was straightforward: Track this new public health threat, identify it, and figure out how to treat it medically. Such actions, however, especially in a brand new policy area such as this, are never so easy. To begin with, how do we know it is a phenomenon that needs to be tracked? The answer is not simple. Sometimes we don't, or at least we don't find out in a timely manner.

In the case of AIDS in the United States, most policy analysts point to the first official indication as occurring on June 5, 1981. This is the date on which the CDC's *Mortality and Morbidity Weekly Report* released a short report stating that five cases of *Pneumocystis carinii* pneumonia (PCP)—a disease that usually occurs only among people with depressed immune systems—had been found in five young previously healthy men in the Los Angeles area.[10] Although the doctors who made the report to the CDC had noted that the men were gay, mention of this characteristic was stripped from the title of the published report for fear that it would raise political problems.[11] This report was followed by a second in July 1981 that noted the occurrence of an unusual form of cancer, Kaposi's sarcoma, in New York City and San Francisco among twenty-six young gay men during the previous thirty months.

Given these reports, it seems logical that the CDC would decide to investigate homosexuality as a factor in the strange phenomenon that was unfolding, and several other factors made it even more likely. One was a hepatitis B study that the CDC had just completed in cooperation with a cluster of gay community health clinics. Among the findings was the significant association of hepatitis B with large numbers of male sexual partners and with anal sexual contact. These findings were bolstered by other studies that showed an increase in the number and variety of sexually transmitted diseases among gay men and linked these increases to gay liberation and its attendant proliferation of sexual institutions.[12]

Although these factors provided the CDC with incentives to investigate the link between gay men and the new syndrome, other factors worked against pursuing other risk groups. By 1982 the CDC had published accounts of the syndrome in heterosexuals of both genders, most of which seemed to be linked to injection drug use, hemophilia, or being from Haiti. Yet the drug use variable, which seemed to be linked to the largest number of nonhomosexual cases, was not pursued as aggressively as the "gay link."

Several factors may account for this disinclination. For one thing, the federal bureaucracy that is empowered to investigate issues related to injection drug use, the National Institute on Drug Abuse (NIDA), emphasizes drug abuse itself rather than diseases that are common to drug users. NIDA therefore chose to leave any investigations of the new disease to researchers in other components of NIH and to the CDC, which unfortunately had little experience and consequently little initiative in dealing with this population.[13] This problem was compounded by the fact that injection drug users are perceived to be a difficult population to study, given their often transient lifestyle (making follow-up difficult) and their fears about the consequences of honestly answering questions about illegal risk activities.

Researchers also have pointed out that in New York City—the most likely area for tracking the "drug connection" because it has the largest estimated population of injection drug users in the country—there were several additional impediments to early recognition of AIDS among injection drug users. They argue that the city's drug treatment system (the institution with the greatest potential for bringing marginalized individuals back into "the system") was not well suited for recognizing and dealing with a new medical condition. Furthermore, professionals within the system had little incentive to change because of the desire to sideline issues that might detract from the primary goal of getting people to stop using illegal drugs.[14]

The tendency to track cases linked to gay sex most aggressively led to at least one red herring along the way, when researchers attempted to link the new syndrome not simply to sexual contact but also to "lifestyle." Having found that many of the early cases among gay men were linked to large numbers of sexual contacts and to recreational drug use, one of the first epidemiological studies examined the use of amyl nitrate ("poppers") as a cause of immunosuppression. A study performed by NIH and the Uniformed Services University of Health Sciences (USUHS) attempted to assess the relationship between Kaposi's sarcoma (a type of skin cancer that showed up in many of the early cases among gay men) and amyl nitrate by comparing two gay men with Kaposi's sarcoma against fifteen healthy gay male volunteers. Despite the small sample numbers, the study concluded that amyl nitrate inhalation might predispose gay men to immune deficiency and further spurred research down the "gay lifestyle" path.[15]

By 1983 the CDC had been able to determine—by tracking individuals within all four of the initial risk groups it identified (Haitians, homosexual men, heroin injectors, and hemophiliacs)—that the immunosuppressive agent appeared to be spread in the same way as hepatitis B (through the exchange of body fluids). Like hepatitis, it would turn out to be linked to a blood-borne virus. The syndrome by this point also had a name—AIDS—to replace terms then being used that linked it only to gay individuals (GRID, gay-related immune deficiency, and KSOI, Kaposi's sarcoma—opportunistic infection). The epidemiological work that went into tracking the syndrome set into motion, however, a dynamic that would result in permanent identification of the gay community with the new disease. According to analyst Steven Epstein, "AIDS became a 'gay disease' primarily because clinicians, epidemiologists, and reporters perceived it through that filter, but secondarily because gay communities were obliged to make it their own."[16]

While epidemiologists were tracking the epidemic, laboratory scientists were attempting to discover the viral agent that the CDC hypothesized was causing the damage. In the United States, credit for the isolation of HIV is given to Dr. Robert Gallo, a researcher within NIH who worked with a class of viruses called retroviruses. Retroviruses, like all viruses, work by infecting cells and causing the cells to produce new viruses according to the genetic code of the virus. Whereas ordinary viruses use their genetic DNA blueprint to produce RNA, which produces proteins that are then assembled into new viruses, retroviruses have another step. They start as RNA and use an enzyme called reverse transcriptase to create DNA; then that DNA moves through the rest of the steps to produce new viruses. Gallo had discovered a class of viruses that are believed to cause cancer, which he named human T-cell leukemia virus (HTLV).

When the initial hypotheses of a lifestyle link were floating around, Gallo saw no link between his research and AIDS. When James Curran of the CDC announced at a meeting of NIH scientists his hypothesis that the syndrome was caused by an infectious agent, however, Gallo began to study the possibility that this agent was a variant of HTLV.[17] At the same time that Gallo was working in the United States, Dr. Luc Montagnier, head of viral oncology at the renowned Pasteur Institute in France, was investigating a retrovirus that killed the T-helper cells that normally help humans mount an immune response to an infection. Montagnier sent Gallo a sample of the virus that he had isolated and named lymphadenopathy-associated virus (LAV).

What happened next remains a matter of controversy to this day. In April 1984, reports began to circulate claiming that Gallo had discovered a new virus, HTLV-III; on April 23, 1984, President Reagan's Secretary of HHS, Margaret Heckler, announced at a press conference that the probable cause of AIDS had been found.[18] Less than a year later, investigators determined that Gallo's virus bore such a strong genetic similarity to Montagnier's that they had to be from the same source. Whether by accident (viral contamination is a continual possibility in viral research) or design, Gallo had called Montagnier's virus his own.[19]

In addition to the never-resolved issue of the origin of Gallo's discovery, the announcement of the virus as the probable causal agent of AIDS paved the way for several other controversies. One of these controversies, which erupted again on an international level in the summer of 2000, came from dissenters to the theory that HIV is, in fact, the cause of AIDS. Some researchers argued (and a few still maintain today) that HIV has never been proven to cause AIDS and that there are other compelling theories that lifestyle or a combination of factors might be at the root of what is, after all, a syndrome (as opposed to a single disease). A second, more practical problem emerged around the question of whether it was better to begin research on drugs that would specifically target HIV or to conduct research on drugs that could be used to combat the problems that occur when a patient's immune system is compromised by HIV.

The HIV-causes-AIDS hypothesis rapidly became widely accepted during the two-year period following the Heckler announcement. Some researchers and patients remained skeptical, however. They based their arguments largely on two lines of thought: a "soft" line dissent and a "hard" line dissent. The soft line dissent does not necessarily believe that there is no link between HIV and AIDS. The soft line argument would be open to the possibility that additional conditions, or cofactors, might be necessary along with HIV to trigger AIDS. One of the most widely circulating variants of the soft view appeared in 1990, when Montagnier supported the 1986 research of a virologist named Shyh-Ching Lo. Lo had discovered the presence of a pathogen called a mycoplasma that he believed might interact with HIV to cause AIDS.

Whereas the soft line view essentially regards HIV as a sort of necessary-but-not-sufficient condition for AIDS to develop, the hard line regards the presence of HIV in someone with immune suppression as extraneous. People who hold this view argue that immune suppression also can occur in people who are not HIV-positive. Most adherents of the hard line approach also support some form of the so-called "risk-AIDS" and "drug-AIDS" hypotheses. These hypotheses suggest that people with immune suppression must belong to some group that is at risk for immune suppression from some lifestyle condition. The most famous proponent of these explanations, Dr. Peter Duesberg, has suggested several explanations for immune suppression in different risk groups. Heavy drug use, including use of injection drugs such as heroin and cocaine and "partying" drugs such as poppers; sexually transmitted diseases, especially among gay men, together with heavy use of antibiotics to treat them; blood transfusion and the use of clotting factor among hemophiliacs and others who need blood products; and, in Africa, extreme malnutrition and lack of sanitation all, according to Duesberg and his adherents, are the real reasons for AIDS symptoms among people who are HIV-infected.[20]

Critics have pointed out several problems with Duesberg's claims. For instance, what can explain the illness and subsequent death of female sexual partners of hemophiliacs who had no known risk factor other than having been infected with HIV by their monogamous male hemophiliac partners? Similarly, how does the risk hypothesis explain the death of infants who got HIV from their mothers? A further development of the Duesberg theory to answer these cases—that azidothymidine (AZT) and other drugs that are used to treat AIDS are themselves immunosuppressive—has been dismissed by many critics as unsatisfying. What, then, would explain immunosuppression in these types of cases before the advent of AZT, or before it had been prescribed to a particular patient?

Ironically, the strongest opponents of the HIV-causes-AIDS assumption (self-proclaimed dissenters, though their critics refer to them as denialists) come from the far left and the far right. In 1990 the Heritage Foundation, a conservative think tank, published a lengthy article written by Duesberg and Bryan J. Ellison in its journal, *Policy Review*.[21] Given Duesberg's theory's regarding the primacy of sexual promiscuity and drug use in causing the symptoms of AIDS, it is hardly surprising that his arguments found a welcome audience among extreme conservatives looking to cut federal spending on AIDS and strongly discourage drug use and sex between men. Adoption of these theories by several renegade chapters of ACT UP is much more perplexing, however. In 1990 ACT UP San Francisco split, to allow members of the original group to concentrate on broader social issues and members of ACT UP Golden Gate to work on treatment and treatment access. ACT UP Golden Gate ultimately became Survive AIDS to avoid any association with the name ACT UP San Francisco, which had experienced an influx of new members and had come to be associated with a denialist perspective. The remaining ACT UP San Francisco and a spin-off, ACT UP Hollywood, have been renounced by other ACT UP chapters, who consider them dangerous and capable of undoing many of the advances of activism by earlier ACT UP chapters. Ironically, the denialist chapters—ACT UP San Francisco in particular—argue that the HIV-causes-AIDS thesis is homophobic because it "demonizes" unprotected sex among men. They also argue that AIDS antiretrovirals are toxic and cause the symptoms of AIDS and that the "AIDS scare" is a scam being perpetrated by profiteering drug companies.

In the summer of 2000, South African president Thabo Mbeki, whose country played host to the Thirteenth International AIDS Conference, gave the denialist camp a boost by openly questioning the link between HIV and AIDS. In addition to empaneling a group of scientists, including Peter Duesberg, to reexamine the issue prior to the conference, in his opening speech at the conference he disappointed scientists worldwide who had hoped he would renounce his questioning of the HIV-causes-AIDS hypothesis. Instead, he alluded to the idea that poverty rather than HIV was the real reason for his nation's suffering, thereby leaving the question open.

In addition to creating a fringe movement of people who did not buy the idea that HIV causes AIDS, widespread propagation of the theory also raised a burning question. Amid an atmosphere of few resources, no time, and frantic patients, everyone treating or being treated for HIV began to ask whether resources would be better spent on finding ways to treat the actual virus or on working with drugs that would treat the conditions caused by the immune suppressing effects of the virus. Two very different perspectives emerged on this issue—breaking down, in large part, along research versus clinical lines.

The position taken by most laboratory researchers—to go with research aimed at the virus itself—had a certain intuitive appeal. After all, now that HIV had been identified, why not go after the root of the problem? A more cynical view was that this approach had the greater career-enhancing potential. The discoverer of a cure for AIDS would be destined for a Nobel prize and the history books. The researcher who discovered that some already-synthesized-and-in-use compound also was able to knock out, say, pneumocystis in AIDS patients would be destined for no such glory and, possibly, not much money either. When HIV was discovered, the field of retrovirology was in its infancy. Thus, the strategy of antiretroviral research for combating AIDS could be characterized as expensive, long-term, and high-risk but with an enormous payoff if successful.

Predictably, people who already were infected and their health care providers were less enthusiastic about this long-term approach. They wanted something more concrete to help with the everyday infections ravaging their bodies. Of course they wanted a cure; they obviously had the most to lose without one. In the meantime, however, they needed treatments to help keep the opportunistic infections at bay. And those treatments had to be affordable and accessible.

This underlying (and sometimes overt) tension between advocates of a long-term antiretroviral research strategy (usually members of the "establishment" research community employed by government and the pharmaceutical industry) and proponents of an expeditious search for treatment of opportunistic infections has had important implications for the development of new treatments. A 1990 article in the *Los Angeles Times* argued that by that point the antiretroviral side clearly had the upper hand in terms of attention and funding but that the tide was slowing and starting to turn, at least in part because of a drug that had been found to stave off attacks of *pneumocystis* pneumonia, a leading killer of people with AIDS.[22] As chapter 2 reveals, this drug—aerosolized pentamidine—was researched largely at the community level by patients and their doctors who were tired of waiting for the government to get around to it.

Resolution of these opening policy controversies over the seemingly straightforward first steps of dealing with a new and deadly syndrome has been anything but simple. In fact, some of them remain ongoing. As with all of the policy areas I examine in the remainder of this book, decisions of the government and larger society about how to begin (let alone complete) the tasks of tracking, identifying, and controlling AIDS have been defined by the opinions and strengths of various groups in and out of government as they struggle to force the policy closer to their own vision.

Policy Dilemma Preview

In the succeeding chapters I examine five AIDS policy areas. Each area has undergone important transformational processes since it was initially formulated. Some policy decisions, such as what groups to study in tracking the epidemic and what types of drugs to study for treating AIDS, were first made at a time when little was known about HIV or AIDS. As the level of our knowledge has increased and as the demographics of the spread of the virus have shifted, many policies have been reexamined. Some actors, such as the pharmaceutical companies, have been through certain battles in multiple stages. For example, the pharmaceutical giant Burroughs Wellcome came under heavy fire when it first released AZT in 1987 for overpricing the drug. Today the same company (except that two mergers later it is part of the even larger Glaxo SmithKline), along with many of its fellow pharmaceutical companies, is undergoing similar pressures, often from the same activists (or sometimes a younger generation of the same groups), but this time the bulk of the controversy is over its pricing policies in developing countries.

Although in this book I have isolated the issues into specific policy areas, it is important to remember that many of them were developed during the same time frames and were worked on by the same actors. For example, AIDS activist groups such as ACT UP often simultaneously worked on campaigns to push for more research into promising drugs, to protest the pricing of drugs already in existence, and to promote sexual education and needle-exchange programs to prevent the spread of HIV. Similarly, the Secretary of HHS is responsible for the health of all Americans and must decide which battles to pick when, at any given time, issues around funding for AIDS medical care, requests for social services for HIV-infected patients and their families, recommendations regarding whether to endorse needle exchange, and a half dozen other AIDS-related policies are all vying for attention and resolution.

Chapter 2 addresses a profound concern of people who have AIDS: medical treatment. As medical treatments began to be developed, patients were concerned that they quickly be made available and affordable. So great was the sense of urgency in this regard that AIDS activists went beyond the boundaries of expected patient behavior to procure drugs by participating heavily in their development, regulation, and pricing. At the same time, they also educated themselves and demanded a new, more powerful role in their own treatment. As drug technology has advanced and the use of multiple antiretroviral medication has become the standard of care, activist patients have again insisted on being part of the decision-making and recommendation process. All of this has forced the traditional policy actors in the area of treatment—government researchers and administrators, medical doctors, and the pharmaceutical industry—to share power (sometimes grudgingly) with people who are HIV-positive and their advocates.

The policy area described in chapter 3, blood policy, disproportionately affects a small group of people. Although anyone could have a blood transfusion, during any given year relatively few people actually do. For those people—and, more crucially, for people who are regular consumers of blood products, particularly people with bleeding disorders such as hemophilia—however, the safety of the blood supply is a life-and-death issue. During the early 1980s, the nonprofit and for-profit sides of the blood industry for several reasons failed to safeguard the blood supply from the threat of viral infection. Chapter 3 addresses why this happened and how those who received contaminated blood and blood products reacted, as well as how these events have shaped the government's current blood policy.

Prevention of further HIV transmission is a profoundly important AIDS policy issue. In chapter 4 I take up the difficult question of how best to achieve the lowest levels of new infections and illness among people who are currently uninfected. In this examination I look at three of the most controversial AIDS prevention policy areas: sex education and condom distribution for adolescents, needle exchange for injection drug users, and mandatory testing of newborn infants. This is an area of AIDS policy in which emotions run very high on all sides, and proposed solutions are about not only the best numerical results but also the values of the communities proposing them.

One of the unique aspects of AIDS is that it has been used to create new demands on government. One of the best examples of this dynamic of new and rising expectations is the establishment of the Ryan White CARE Act, which is the subject of chapter 5. Enacted in 1990, this Act is a piece of landmark legislation in the sense that it was the first time government created a new national system of services for a particular disease. Because it was designed to be reauthorized every five years, it has become a window into the shifting issues and demographics of AIDS in the United States. During its enactment as well as with its two reauthorizations thus far, groups have pitted themselves against one another—cities versus states, some cities versus other cities, gay-based organizations against ones founded within minority communities—as all seek to make the case that they are most deserving of the considerable resources the government is distributing.

The final policy area I examine in the book has only recently emerged as an area of concern for the United States, although it had reached crisis proportions years previously. That issue area, U.S. foreign policy regarding AIDS in developing countries, particularly in sub-Saharan Africa, is the subject of chapter 6. Resolutions of the questions of how much the United States should do, what should be done, and where the government should position itself in controversies between U.S.-based private companies and African governments will have profound effects on the lives of tens of millions of people living in many of the world's poorest countries.

One of the challenges of understanding AIDS policy is that it is a rapidly moving target. In fewer than twenty years, the United States has gone from not even having a name for the syndrome to spending billions of dollars on it in a multitude of programs that never were envisioned for any other type of illness. Yet AIDS is more than just a policy area that is unique for its rapid explosion as an issue into the policy arena. It also is important for its spillover effects into other policy areas, as well as into relationships between governments and citizens and between for-profit corporations and governments. Furthermore, the policy contests around specific topics also are representative of more general dynamics. AIDS treatment and prevention questions turn on more general and unresolved values debates. Blood policy is as much about the important and common policy tool of regulation as is it about the specific dilemmas involved in maintaining a blood supply that is safe and plentiful. The Ryan White CARE Act is a landmark piece of legislation in one sense but an utterly typical one in the sense that, like many before or since, it seeks to redistribute benefits among competing groups. The dilemmas that surround AIDS as a foreign policy issue reflect our country's general unresolved dilemmas about membership, or who deserves to take part in the distribution of resources. To understand how AIDS policy has been developed and is continuing to be developed—with many actors involved in the competitions toward policy outcomes and many facets of policy being worked on at any given moment—is to go a long way toward understanding the policy process for any issue.

CHAPTER 2

New Drugs, New Rules, New Relationships

On March 24, 1987, ACT UP/New York (the first of the ACT UP chapters that would spread across the country) conducted its first protest. More than 250 members of the new organization participated in a demonstration on Wall Street. The main target of the protest was the pharmaceutical company Burroughs Wellcome, which had set the price of AZT, its newly approved antiretroviral drug, at $10,000 for a year's supply. AZT was the first drug licensed specifically as an anti-HIV drug; although its critics and even many of its proponents warned that it had major limitations and side effects, it was hailed by many desperate consumers and their treatment providers as the source of hope they had been waiting for. Thus, it seemed to be a particularly cruel irony that the long-awaited treatment should be priced out of the reach of many people who sought it.

Many features of ACT UP's first demonstration would become standard operating procedure for others that followed. The protesters brought all kinds of useful props with them: an effigy of FDA Commissioner Frank Young, copies of an op-ed piece that had been written by activist Larry Kramer and published in the *New York Times* the day before, and fact sheets bearing the headline "AIDS is everybody's business now." Although the primary target was Burroughs Wellcome and its perceived profiteering, ACT UP also used its forum-for-the-day to take on the FDA (which the group accused of colluding with Burroughs Wellcome and moving too slowly in approving other drugs), NIH (which it accused of conducting "inhumane" clinical trials), the insurance industry (for denying benefits to people with, or at risk for, AIDS), and the president (for failing to acknowledge the epidemic).[1]

The catchy slogans, fact sheets, and targeting of multiple enemies were not the only precedent-setting tactics of this first big event. The action also was the first of many that were destined to disrupt business as usual (tying up traffic for hours), get people arrested (seventeen, in this case), and make the national news. By the end of the day, the country had been put on notice that a new group of actors would be contributing to the decisions being made about AIDS policy.

Four years earlier, an action of another sort had taken place.[2] In that case, there were no arrests, although there was a deliberately planned disruption and a dramatic pronouncement. The setting was the second AIDS Forum in Denver, Colorado; the year was 1983; and the actors were self-proclaimed people with AIDS (PWAs). About a dozen PWAs, who had made the individual decision to attend the conference to be sure their ideas and interests would be directly represented, had assembled in a hospitality suite that had been set aside for them. As they compared notes, they discovered that all of them had been subject to similar patronizing treatment, and they decided to act. Two PWAs, Michael Callen and Bobbi Campbell, were appointed to give voice to their collective discontent.

They chose to create a manifesto of sorts: an enumeration for PWAs, the public at large, and health care professionals of how PWAs ought to be treated. These principles, many of which strongly resembled ideas from the women's health movement of previous decades, all promoted ideas of self-empowerment—beginning with the notion that people who are sick from AIDS should be referred to as neither "victims" nor "patients" but "people with AIDS." There were seventeen principles in all. They were unveiled with much fanfare when the PWA group stormed the forum's closing session, unfurled their banner proclaiming "Fighting for our Lives," and took turns reading the individual points of what was to become known collectively as the Denver Principles.

The self-empowerment and activism that these actions exemplify are important because they challenge a common perception most of us have about the way in which drugs are developed and approved in the United States. Drug development is not an objective, isolated process. Although scientists in white lab coats figure prominently, so do activists dressed in black t-shirts and politicians trying to balance the demands of their constituents with the arguments of industries that contribute to their campaigns. Decisions about which drugs get developed, how they are discovered and tested, what price tags they are given, and who decides who should take them are political and are determined, like other AIDS policies, by political struggles.

Although these struggles are decidedly political, they also, of course, revolve around scientific findings and differing interpretations of those findings. This dynamic creates a policy situation that is complicated to highly trained individuals, let alone the casual observer. Providing a comprehensive look at all of the developments in treatment policy since the late 1980s is beyond the scope of this book. A much more manageable option—and the one I take—is to use important examples to illustrate consistent themes in the struggles surrounding treatment policies. The remainder of the chapter is devoted to three specific topics. First, I look at the development of the first and most famous antiretroviral drug, AZT. Then I examine the case of aerosolized pentamidine, a drug that was widely used to treat AIDS patients before antiretroviral treatments become available. Finally, I look at the development of the self-empowerment model of treatment and its current impact in a world with many more treatment options than when it was developed.

For Every Solution, a New Problem: The Case of AZT

Policy making often is represented as an exercise in finding the right solution to a given problem. As chapter 1 suggests, however, the "right" solution depends in very large part on who is defining the problem. The "right solution" debate between people who advocated an antiviral approach and those who proposed intensive research into opportunistic infections was further accelerated by the development of the first FDA-approved drug for the treatment of HIV infection, AZT. AZT's development was fraught with controversy, and that controversy only increased once the final product was approved. It was hailed by some people as a miracle drug that would transform AIDS from a rapidly fatal disease to a chronic disease ("until the cure—there's Retrovir") and by others as a poorly tested, toxic drug whose profit-generating capacity far exceeded its usefulness as a medical therapy.

The development of AZT also demonstrates just how hazy the line between public and private policy really is. Technically, the drug was developed by a private actor (the pharmaceutical giant Burroughs Wellcome), but its development was heavily dependent on government actors throughout the process. From the use of government-funded labs in the early stages of research to the FDA's oversight of the clinical trials the drug went through, the work of the government was an integral part of AZT's development. Later, when AIDS patients and their allies were angered at the prices being charged for AZT, they worked to bring the government back into the process—this time in the form of members of Congress, asking in place of their constituents on what basis Burroughs Wellcome was setting its prices. Later still, as more studies and other treatment options became available, some activists openly questioned the government's acceptance of pharmaceutical claims about the many benefits that AZT could provide.

Before the advent of AZT, treatment professionals were limited to treating the opportunistic infections that manifested themselves in HIV-positive individuals. They commonly resorted to drugs already in existence for treating such infections. Prior to the advent of AIDS, researchers had discovered that people whose immune systems were purposely suppressed for the purpose of receiving transplanted organs or who had experienced immunity-compromising chemotherapy had similar opportunistic infections, and community doctors used the same treatments for the new set of patients.

The April 23, 1984, announcement by HHS Secretary Margaret Heckler, that the virus that causes AIDS had been discovered dramatically changed things. With a tangible viral enemy before them, researchers now had a target for new drug development, and they enthusiastically set themselves to the task. Burroughs Wellcome already had a hand in the treatment of AIDS-related opportunistic infections. The company held the patents on Septra, which was used to treat PCP, and Zovirax, which was used to treat the herpes infections that often went from latent to active form in HIV-positive patients.[3] Several weeks after the Heckler announcement, Burroughs Wellcome went to work directly on an antiretroviral agent.

As the pharmaceutical industry is fond of pointing out, the costs for developing new drugs can be high. The process for getting drugs approved also can be time-consuming. At the time AZT was being developed, a drug typically took an average of eight years from the initiation of clinical trials to FDA approval.[4] The quickest and cheapest way to find a "new" drug is to rediscover an already-synthesized compound that has the properties being sought for a particular condition. In the case of AIDS, this meant running various chemical compounds in tests with the live virus and seeing if antiviral activity occurred in the test tube (in scientific terms, *in vitro*).

There was an additional problem for the pharmaceutical labs contemplating the challenge of finding an anti-HIV drug: the danger in the lab area itself. HIV research had to be conducted in the most secure lab setting, dictating what is known as a P-3 level of biosafety. The labs that Burroughs Wellcome was using were not set up at this high level, so it, like many other labs, shipped compounds to labs at Duke University, the FDA, and the National Cancer Institute (NCI). There, research teams had offered to run various tests to determine the antiviral activity of potential drugs.[5] Each of the potential drugs sent out by Burroughs Wellcome had been alphabetically coded, and two of the three labs found that Compound S, azidothymidine, was active against live HIV in the test tube.[6]

When Burroughs Wellcome got the good news from the labs at Duke and NCI, it quickly started the ball rolling on the approval process. David Barry, a former FDA researcher who had become a virologist at Burroughs Wellcome, called Ellen Cooper, head of the Division of Antiviral Drug Products at the FDA. He asked if they could expedite the process in getting AZT classified as an investigational new drug (IND). Cooper suggested that Burroughs Welcome send in all the information it had so far, so that she would have already read most of the data when the final application was completed and sent. Barry complied, and when the final full application was sent, Cooper took less than a week to grant Wellcome an IND designation for AZT.[7]

The quick IND response was the first step in a long process. Although there now are some expedited processes in place, traditionally FDA regulations provide for a three-phase set of tests before the agency considers approval of any drug. Phase I is required to certify the safety of the drug. In addition to the question of whether the drug is toxic, Phase I trials are used to decide how the drug should be given and in what dosage. Phase I trials are relatively short (usually less than a year) and involve only a few patients.

Phase II trials are designed to measure a drug's efficacy (that is, whether it actually works). Phase II also is used to confirm the safety findings of Phase I, more precisely define the best dosage, and make comparisons to similar drugs. These trials involve more patients than Phase I (but usually fewer than 200) and typically take about three years.

Phase III trials are large scale, involving up to several thousand patients, and long term, usually requiring one to three years. They confirm the findings of the earlier trials and look at long-term results of the drug use.

When Phase III is finished, a new drug application (NDA) is submitted to the FDA. The NDA contains an analysis of all data collected and may be thousands of pages long. The FDA reviews the application and may require new data or more analysis of existing data. If the FDA approves the drug, the pharmaceutical company is free to begin marketing and distributing the product.

Phase I trials for AZT began on July 3, 1985, with nineteen subjects at two sites: the NCI's clinic in Bethesda, Maryland, and Duke University. The trial ran for six weeks and offered hopeful but ambiguous conclusions. The researchers noted, "some of the patients treated with AZT improved over the six weeks." They could not say, however, whether the improvements would be sustained, whether AZT therapy could be tolerated by people undergoing it, whether viral drug resistance might occur, and most important, "ultimately, whether AZT will affect disease progression or survival."[8]

In February 1986, Phase II trials began at Duke and NCI.[9] These trials had 282 subjects, although only 27 of them participated in all twenty-four weeks of the study. The trial was described as placebo-controlled and double-blind. This means that half the patients received the placebo, and neither the doctors nor the patients knew who was getting the AZT. From a research perspective, placebo-controlled, double-blind trials are considered the "cleanest," yielding the best results the most quickly. From the perspective of AIDS activists, the placebo-controlled, double-blind trial symbolizes everything that is needlessly cruel and out-of-touch with reality in the academic realm.

This first experience with AZT provided much of the activist critique of early clinical trials. Activists objected to the idea of withholding a potentially useful drug from half of the group studied, as well as the strict criteria that researchers had set up for entrance into the study in the first place. (Participants were excluded if they had taken almost any other recent drug treatments.)[10] They also argued the impossibility of keeping a trial double-blind, and the experience of AZT proved them right.

One of the most outspoken critics of AZT as a drug therapy, John Lauritsen, quotes Ellen Cooper as conceding that "the fact that the treatment groups unblinded themselves early could have resulted in bias in the workup of the patients."[11] Although the trial investigators claimed that "the placebo was indistinguishable from the AZT and similar in taste,"[12] Lauritsen quotes Cooper in noting that this was not the case in the early part of the trial; he further argues that some trial subjects had their pills chemically analyzed, and others pooled and shared their medications to increase the odds that all might get the drug. He also contends that the trials were further unblinded from the perspective of the attending investigators. Because AZT had extreme effects on the blood profiles of patients taking it, the blood profiles of patients' charts signaled to the researchers who was on the drug.

Despite the many problems with the study, investigators were able to report one widely circulated conclusion: Twenty-four weeks into the study, nineteen subjects in the placebo group and only one in the AZT group had died. In September 1986 the trial was officially halted, and the placebo patients were offered the drug.

Although testing continued, Burroughs Wellcome was allowed to waive the requirement of a Phase III trial and instead concentrate on its NDA, which it submitted in piecemeal fashion between October and December 1986.[13] An FDA advisory meeting was held on January 16, 1987, and the committee voted ten to one to recommend the drug. The FDA adopted the committee's recommendation in March 1987, and Burroughs Wellcome began marketing. During the interim between testing and final approval, Burroughs Wellcome provided 4,500 patients with the drug free of charge under a treatment IND program—a provision the company was quick to note in justifying the price of AZT to Congress.

The price originally set for AZT, approximately $10,000 for a year's supply, caught PWAs and their advocates by surprise. During a congressional hearing on March 10, 1987, devoted entirely to the subject, the chief executive officer (CEO) of Burroughs Wellcome, T. E. Haigler, Jr., offered an extensive laundry list of factors that normally go into any drug pricing decision. He also argued that material costs in this case were particularly high and that there were uncertainties regarding the market, the usefulness of AZT, and the advent of other new therapies that all necessitated the price tag the company had selected.

Congressman Henry Waxman, a California representative who had initiated this set of hearings and whose constituency had been strongly affected by AIDS, was unconvinced by the argument. Viewing the market for the drug, he estimated that, at $10,000 a person, simply supplying AZT to people using the drug under the treatment IND would net the company $45 million in the first year. If AZT were supplied to all 25,000 Americans estimated to be infected by the end of 1987, that projection, he noted, would move to $250 million.

A like-minded colleague, Representative Ron Wyden (D-Ore.), joined Waxman in his quest for specific numbers from the company regarding how much the drug had cost to develop and how much the company believed it would make. When Burroughs Wellcome refused to divulge the numbers, Wyden asked the CEO a final question that revealed the level of his cynicism: "Why didn't you set the price at $100,000 per patient?"[14]

When the FDA announced its approval of AZT on March 19, 1987, and Burroughs Wellcome unveiled its $10,000 price tag, activists took to the streets. This announcement galvanized the Wall Street protest by the infant ACT UP against Burroughs Wellcome and various other creators of AIDS policy.

Burroughs Wellcome did lower the annual cost of the drug from $10,000 to $8,000, but this controversy was destined to be only the first in a series of struggles over what the appropriate cost and uses of the drug should be. By fall 1989 AZT was still the only drug licensed to directly treat the AIDS virus, but several research findings had worked to expand the drug's market. The first study, ACTG 019, concluded that people with HIV infection could benefit from AZT therapy to delay the onset of full-blown AIDS. Because AZT previously had been recommended only for patients with an AIDS diagnosis, this finding created an increase of more than tenfold in the potential market.[15] At the same time, a treatment for the most common opportunistic infection associated with AIDS, pneumocystis pneumonia, had been developed, thereby prolonging the lives and, by extension, AZT use, of AIDS patients.[16]

Initially, Burroughs Wellcome had rejected the demands of AIDS advocacy groups to lower AZT's price in the face of these developments.[17] Neither AIDS activists nor their allies took the news lying down, however. In 1989 the *New York Times* editorialized:

> Burroughs at first justified its astoundingly high price for AZT by noting rival drugs would soon be on the market. But the rival drugs still haven't appeared. Burroughs did reduce the retail price from $10,000 to $8,000 in 1987. The company now says the present 40,000 AIDS patients are the only customers it can be sure of. Every epidemiologist expects the toll to rise higher.[18]

On September 14, 1989, ACT UP/New York publicized the arguments of the *New York Times* editorial with a new dramatic action. Five protesters led the way by faking their way into the New York Stock Exchange, unfurling a banner proclaiming "Sell Wellcome," and using foghorns to stop transactions for five minutes.

When the protesters were arrested and taken away, 1,500 ACT UP activists took up the fight outside with foghorns, placards, and leaflets.[19] Other ACT UP groups in London and San Francisco held demonstrations on the same day, and activists began a boycott and public information campaign (mainly in the form of affixing "AIDS Profiteer" labels) against Burroughs Wellcome over-the counter-products, including Sudafed, Actifed, and Neosporin. Confronted with these mounting protests, Burroughs Wellcome backed down, and on September 18, 1989, it announced a 20 percent price cut, bringing a full-dose year's supply (patients who did not have full-blown AIDS were on a lesser dosage) to approximately $6,500 per year.[20]

The fall in AZT's price presaged a decline in the drug's reputation in succeeding years. Almost from the beginning, activists argued about the value of AZT. Predictably, fringe AIDS denialists denounced it as worthless. After all, if HIV doesn't cause AIDS, who needs a drug to combat HIV? The fact that Burroughs Wellcome donated money to several mainstream and radical AIDS groups also helped to foster the impression that potential detractors might be allowing themselves to be "bought off."[21]

In 1993, new evidence from a preliminary report on the European Concorde study cast doubt on the wisdom of AZT as an early intervention. This study featured more than 1,500 participants who were randomly selected to go into the treatment group, where they received 1,000 mg of AZT daily, or the placebo group, where they were given a placebo unless and until they showed symptoms of AIDS, at which point they were given AZT.[22] The study ran for three years, making it the longest study of its kind, and it generated waves of defensive press in the United States. According to the Concorde study, the experimental group did show a rise in counts of a type of blood cell known as CD4 cells (sometimes also called T-cells), just as they had in ACTG 019. There were no significant differences between the two groups, however, in three-year survival rates, rate of disease progression, or development of opportunistic infection.

The Concorde study left researchers scrambling to refute its claims—usually by finding fault with the methodology or interpretation of the study. Many activists also had been dealt a harsh blow by the study, not simply because it questioned the use of a drug that many were relying on heavily but also because it undermined a major activist gain—the use of surrogate markers. Among the many objections that activists had to the way early clinical trials were designed was that they had a particularly nasty way of determining whether a drug worked: whether the patient died. Arguing that trial participants shouldn't have to die for the sake of science, activists had argued for using certain health indicators, or surrogate markers, as a different way of judging how well a drug was doing. Researchers had found that a decline in the level of CD4 cells usually accompanied progression to AIDS. Therefore, activists reasoned that CD4 counts would be a logical, and certainly more humane, way of judging whether a drug was working. In fact, the second anti-HIV medication approved by the FDA, ddI, won its approval in 1991 on the basis of studies that used CD4 counts as surrogate markers. The Concorde study, however, called into question just how important the elevated CD4 counts in the treatment group could be as an indicator, given that there were no significant long-term differences in survival rates or disease progression between the treatment and placebo groups. In other words, if CD4 counts increased in the treatment group but overall survival rates did not, were CD4 counts really indicating anything important?

A few months after Wellcome's price cut, researchers announced that AZT's benefits could be achieved at much lower dosages.[23] Despite its toxicity problems, AZT has had staying power—as demonstrated by the part it often plays in the current tripartite "AIDS cocktail" standard of care. Still, it no longer holds the "best and only hope" status it once held in the late 1980s.

The story of AZT is important for more than its uses in drug therapy, however. The drug's place in history as a political success story for activists seeking changes in experimental drug policy is clear. AZT was a pathbreaking drug not only in clinical terms but also because of its mobilizing effects. During the course of AZT's trials and the first few years of its marketing, patients and their allies discovered that they had power, individually and as a group. People previously classified only as "experimental subjects" made individual decisions (like having their pills analyzed and sharing pills) that bucked medical authority, and consumers, as a group, mobilized themselves to successfully fight a pricing structure that seemed to be unchangeable (given that Burroughs Wellcome had a monopoly on antiretrovirals at the time).

The AZT story also offers more general policy insights. One is that what sometimes looks like a policy solution (such as finding a desperately needed medication) can easily be recast as a policy problem (such as when the price is considered too high). The AZT experience also demonstrates that government can work to the advantage of the private sector (for example, by expediting a drug approval process) and grassroots community activists (for example, by holding embarrassing hearings on pricing policies). Such decisions, however, are based not only (and in some cases, only marginally) on the merits of taking action. They usually are a function of the level of organization of the groups and policy advocates involved and the resources these groups have at their disposal.

An "End Run around Federal Incompetence": The Case of Aerolized Pentamidine

As AZT was making its comparatively rapid way through the approval process, community doctors were continuing to treat the opportunistic infections that continued to take the lives of their patients. Not surprisingly, they and their patients had begun to raise questions about why these conditions were not being given similarly high priority. Perhaps the most well-known example was PCP.

Particularly in the early days of the AIDS epidemic, PCP was the leading killer among HIV-infected patients in the United States.[24] Although patients usually survived their initial bout with the pneumonia, subsequent infections left the lungs increasingly damaged, and the third or fourth rounds usually were deadly. Several drugs, including pentamidine in injectable form and the sulfa-based drugs Bactrim and Septra, had been documented as effective treatments for PCP in immunocompromised individuals before the onset of AIDS.[25] Community doctors who knew this put their patients on a treatment (or sometimes, prevention) regimen that was based on one or more of these drugs. Because a very high percentage of these patients had severe reactions to the sulfa-based drugs, pentamidine was an important component of the treatment strategy.

Prior to the advent of AIDS the use of pentamidine had been so rare that the CDC handled any requests for it. The drug was flown from England to the CDC, then sent out on a "compassionate use" (that is, free) basis to the physician requesting it. With the outbreak of the AIDS epidemic, there was a sudden surge in demand. By the end of 1983 there had been more than 2,000 requests, and the CDC was worried that the demand would soon outstrip the supply. In an attempt to avert such a problem, the CDC went shopping for a U.S. drug company that was willing to produce large quantities of injectable pentamidine.

A small company named Lymphomed agreed to supply the CDC with vials of the drug, and soon the CDC was urging Lymphomed to assume total responsibility for making and distributing it. Previously Lymphomed had been primarily a generic drug firm; like all of the firms the CDC had approached, it was wary of sinking resources into a drug with a limited market. The company's decision to go where others had feared to tread has been retrospectively attributed to two very different motivations.

The case for the first motivation, altruism, was put forth by Brian Tambi, Lymphomed's vice president for corporate development, who testified before Congress waving a letter from the National Organization for Rare Disorders that touted Lymphomed as an "outstanding model for the pharmaceutical industry for the development of orphan drugs."[26] The letter went on to acknowledge Lymphomed's courage for being "willing to adopt pentamidine at a time when no one was able to predict the scope of the AIDS epidemic."

An alternative theory about Lymphomed's motivation was quickly suggested by Representative Ted Weiss (D-N.Y.), who opened the committee's questioning. He suggested that the company had gone into pentamidine production as a way to transform a small company on the back of a single product:

> It boggles the mind that you would do that [hire a huge sales force] when you have one product. That's it. You have one product and you go ahead and create a national distribution system of this kind? My sense of it is that you saw a good thing which could be used to build your company to a size that you'd never anticipated. And how do you pay for it? By soaking the clientele.[27]

The inducements to Lymphomed to become the supplier of pentamidine certainly had been made stronger by the passage of the Orphan Drug Act the previous year. This law encouraged drug manufacturers to develop drugs for diseases that were so rare that there is no reasonable expectation that research and development costs will pay off. Among the perks of the orphan drug designation are seven-year exclusive marketing rights on the new drug, research grants, and tax credits for the company developing the drug.

Lymphomed applied for orphan drug status for pentamidine, and injectable pentamidine became the first drug targeted at AIDS patients to receive approval under this designation. This was not the end of the pentamidine saga, however. Although pentamidine might be the drug of choice for treating pneumocystis pneumonia, injection clearly was not the best way of getting the drug into the lungs, where the damage was being done. Moreover, nearly half of the patients who were injected with the drug were having toxic reactions to it.[28] The answer, which already was being toyed with in animal studies, was to aerolize the drug into a mist that could be inhaled directly into the lungs.[29] Word spread quickly among AIDS patients and doctors in New York City. Soon, for patients who were lucky enough to have doctors "in the know," aerolized pentamidine became the standard of care not only for treating bouts of pneumonia but also for preventing their occurrence in the first place. Although only injectable pentamidine had been formally approved by the FDA, community doctors who were treating patients with the aerolizable form were not breaking the law. They were engaging in the common practice of "off–label use": prescribing an FDA-approved drug for a purpose or in a way other than the one listed on the label.

In effect, there was a disparity in treatment: Patients who were well connected and informed (usually gay white men living in urban areas) had access to a life-saving therapy that others (people of color, rural patients) did not enjoy. In fact, the prominent gay New York city-based activist Michael Callen decided to launch the crusade for aerolized pentamidine when he discovered that "poster boy" hemophiliac Ryan White's own physician did not know about aerolized pentamidine. In May 1987, Callen went to the head of the NIAID, Anthony Fauci, and asked him to release guidelines instructing physicians with patients at high risk for PCP to treat it preventively with aerolized pentamidine. Fauci refused, claiming he did not have sufficient evidence on the effectiveness of such treatment to support the issuance of guidelines—in spite of the fact that less than three months earlier, a subcommittee within NIAID had recommended that trials of aerolizable pentamidine be given the highest priority.[30]

Disgusted activists and community doctors had had enough. They knew that aerolized pentamidine was an effective treatment for PCP and, more important, preventing HIV-infected patients from getting the pneumonia in the first place. What they needed was to prove what had already become common knowledge. From this necessity they turned to a radically different type of drug trial: the community-based trial. Rather than leaving it to the government or the private sector to study the effects of aerolized pentamidine, they studied the effects themselves.

The first community-based trial for an unapproved AIDS drug was conducted between July 1, 1987, and December 31, 1988, by the San Francisco County Community Consortium.[31] The study involved 408 participants at twelve sites in the San Francisco area who were randomly assigned to receive one of three dosages: 30 milligrams of aerolized pentamidine every two weeks, 150 milligrams every two weeks, or 300 milligrams every two weeks. Significantly, the community trials dispensed with two controversial elements of many clinical trials. They were not doubleblind and they did not use placebos; in this experiment, everyone got some amount of the drug on trial.

New York City had its own version of the County Community Consortium, the Community Research Initiative. Like its San Francisco counterpart, the

Community Research Initiative reacted to Fauci's refusal to tell doctors to use aerolized pentamidine, and it set up a second community trial patterned after San Francisco's.[32] Although the NIAID had expressed tentative interest in the San Francisco trial, it ultimately decided not to fund it, leaving both community-based networks scrambling for sponsors. In both cases, the largest sponsor ultimately was the pharmaceutical company Lymphomed.

Lymphomed was experiencing its own problems at this point. It had suffered a major blow when the FDA had decided that Lymphomed's exclusive rights on injectable pentamidine did not extend to an aerolizable version. The situation was worsened when another company, Fisons, announced in October 1987 that it would go after the rights on the aerolizable form. Although both companies received initial orphan designation, they would have to, in effect, race to see who would get final approval and exclusive marketing rights for seven years.

Of course, the drug companies and AIDS activists looked at the trials of aerolized pentamidine in very different ways. From the drug company perspective, the race for final orphan drug status was a zero-sum game. One company would get exclusive marketing rights, and the other would lose whatever resources it had sunk into research and development. Activists with AIDS had their own view of the winners-and-losers scenario. For them, winners got access to the drug during this race, and losers died for the want of it. Not surprisingly, these two versions of a high-stake struggle led to some major conflicts.

Generally speaking, the activists cast their lot with Lymphomed. After all, they were working closely with the company in the groundbreaking trials in San Francisco and New York City. This choice did not preclude them, however, from also getting what they could from Fisons during the trial period. ACT UP Boston "zapped" Fisons (located in Bedford, Massachusetts) in August 1988 with a staged funeral and in subsequent meetings with corporate officials from Fisons demanded that the company provide information on where its clinical trials were being conducted and the dosage, timing, and type of nebulizer being tested. They also wanted eligibility criteria for participation in the trials loosened. Fisons ultimately gave in on some counts, agreeing to provide trial site information and some interim nebulizer data.

Lymphomed and Fisons both submitted trial proposal designs to the NIAID in October 1987; what followed was a convoluted trail of disagreements over technical issues, more negotiations, consultations with experts, and further revisions. Finally, the NIAID began enrollment in three trials proposed by Lymphomed (one for treatment, two for prevention) in March and June 1988, after the community trials in San Francisco and New York City were already well under way.

The organizations responsible for drug testing were treated by and reacted to AIDS activists in different ways. Lymphomed found itself collaborating with them to expedite evidence of aerolized pentamidine's effectiveness, and Fisons engaged in damage control to quiet them down. On the government level, public administrators from NIH went on the defensive in trying to answer charges leveled at them by members of Congress who had heard from AIDS activists within their constituencies. These members of Congress wanted to know why NIH hadn't taken the lead in testing aerolizable pentamidine.

During the same set of hearings in which Lymphomed was blasted for its profiteering motives, NIAID head Anthony Fauci also was grilled. Representative Waxman charged that the agency's own drug selection committee had placed the highest priority on testing pentamidine a full thirteen months earlier, yet all that had happened was that three trials had been designed, but no patients had been enrolled in any actual study by NIH.[33]

Fauci defended his agency's inaction, arguing that getting aerolized pentamidine into a trial sooner would have required a staff member whose time was dedicated entirely to that project and that the agency was too short-staffed to dedicate such a position. A second representative, Nancy Pelosi (D-Calif.), jumped on the consequences of the delay, however. She argued that in her hometown of San Francisco it would now be impossible to do the research precisely because no one would be crazy enough to sit around waiting for a trial when they already knew that aerolized pentamidine worked. Rather than volunteer as a trial participant, anyone at risk for pneumonia would be treated with aerolized pentamidine. Thus, trials would be impossible to conduct for lack of participants. Fauci found this point impossible to dispute.

Based on the research that was conducted in collaboration with community-based researchers in San Francisco and New York City, Lymphomed ultimately received the license for aerolized pentamidine. The company's collaboration with activists in research did not extend to pricing, however, and Lymphomed once again found itself on the defensive against activists and their congressional allies.

In October 1984, when Lymphomed had received orphan drug status from the FDA for the injectable form of pentamidine, its had set the wholesale price for a 300 milligram vial (a one-month supply) at $25. As progress with pentamidine moved progressively upward, so did the price. By August 1987, the same vial of pentamidine cost $99.45—a fourfold increase in three years.[34] In testimony before Congress, Lymphomed called the price increase inevitable and claimed that it was justified by the need for a small company to grow to handle an unexpectedly large job. That answer satisfied neither activists nor their congressional advocates. Members of Congress responded rhetorically for the record. Activists, on the other hand, voted with their feet. They took action through the PWA Health Group—the largest buyers' club in the country.

The buyers clubs were created as largely underground organizations that were dedicated to funneling AIDS drugs to AIDS patients. According to one description, they operate "in a shadowy twilight zone somewhere between a licensed drugstore and a pharmaceutical Casbah."[35] On the legitimate side of the ledger are the vitamins, food supplements, and over-the-counter treatments they sell at the lowest possible prices. The underground side of their activities includes importation of drugs that are unavailable or unapproved in the United States.

In September 1989, the New York City-based PWA Health Group issued a public slap in the face to Lymphomed by announcing at a press conference that it would begin importing pentamidine from England because it could get the drug for a fraction of the price at which it was being sold in the United States. This action marked the first organized effort by a buyers' club to import an already-approved medication solely because of cost (as opposed to availability). Lymphomed refused to lower its price. The company argued, as it had earlier, that it needed to recover high research, development, and marketing costs.

The real impact of the buyers' club became evident several years later. In September 1989 Fujisawa, one of Japan's largest pharmaceutical companies, bought Lymphomed and perpetuated the policy of refusing to lower pentamidine's price. As buyers' clubs continued to buy from England (and expanded to Germany as well), Fujisawa hatched a scheme that, according to an internal memo, was designed to recoup the market share that had been lost to the importers.[36] The plan, which was set into motion in December 1989 and January 1990, created a scam "post-marketing study," supposedly designed to determine the effectiveness of varying doses of pentamidine. The "study" was presented to doctors with large AIDS practices by sales representatives who told them they could buy vials at a two-for-one cost if they participated in the study. Fujisawa did not seek FDA approval for the study, as regulation of a legitimate study would dictate; obtain approval from an institutional review board looking at the ethics of the study; or obtain informed consent from those who would be participating. The "study" was shut down without ever gaining any information eight weeks after it was initiated. The company claimed that the study had become "too unwieldy to administer." A more likely explanation is that Fujisawa's thinly veiled marketing attempt backfired. Doctors approached by the company had smelled a rat, and one of them, New York City physician Howard Grossman, blew the whistle on the operation. Buyers' clubs and advocacy groups were publicly scandalized, and Fujisawa's marketing attempts were set back more than ever.

The struggles over the development, testing, distribution, and pricing of aerolized pentamidine contributed a great deal to the overall development of national policies dealing with new pharmaceutical products. Three major groups of actors were involved: activists who were infected and affected by AIDS; private pharmaceutical companies that were trying to quickly and profitably develop a new product; and the federal government, in the form of policymaking agencies such as the FDA and NIH and members of Congress advocating for their constituents. From an activist viewpoint, the failure to develop an efficient and affordable treatment in a timely manner was caused by the usual problems stemming from policies designed by the other two sets of actors (the government and the pharmaceutical industry). First, although pneumocystis was the leading cause of death among PWAs, it was an opportunistic infection, and the priority of researchers in the government and private industry was to develop antiretrovirals. Enrollments in clinical trials established under the old policies were hampered by what the activist community regarded as unnecessary and even dangerous rules, such as the use of placebos after the word was out that aerolized pentamidine clearly worked. Even after aerolized pentamidine had become an approved commonplace treatment, there was no mechanism for keeping the price of the treatment affordable for patients who needed it.

The new policies created by the aerolized pentamidine experience came about in response to these criticisms. Often the changes were instituted at a nongovernmental level and later adopted as official when activists proved that they worked. Frustrated by NIH's refusal to issue treatment guidelines, activists spread the word themselves on the effectiveness of aerolized pentamidine. Angered by NIH's foot-dragging in conducting clinical trials, they created community-based groups to run the trials themselves. Unconvinced that placebos, double-blinding, and strict eligibility rules for who could participate in trials equaled good science, they designed their own trials and produced evidence that was praised by the FDA. Worried that their efforts would be for naught if poor PWAs could not afford aerolized pentamidine once it was approved, they found alternative affordable supplies. In the words of activist Michael Callen, "The AIDS community has done an end-run around federal incompetence and indifference."[37] He might well have added, accurately, that the community had won a struggle to get rid of policies that it considered to be at odds with the goals of PWAs and substituted others in their place.

In the struggle over policy, the outcome often is determined by the relative power of groups engaged in the struggle. In this case, the activist community increased its power through the struggle itself. With aerolized pentamidine, activists demonstrated that PWAs also were potential voters, trial participants, and consumers with corresponding political, scientific, and economic power that they would not hesitate to use to get the drugs they needed. As in the AZT experience, activists achieved policy victories in drug pricing and accessibility. They also legitimized (mainly through the community-based research concept) the role of AIDS patients and their advocates as not simply activist consumers (though this achievement was no small feat) but also as alternative treatment providers. In biological terms, access to aerolized pentamidine has meant the difference between life and death to many people. In policy terms, that same access has meant a major challenge to the way policymakers approach drug pricing and access.

Not Victims, Not Patients, But People with AIDS

The struggles over the development, approval, and pricing of AZT and pentamidine created very visible policy consequences. At the same time, however, a more subtle but equally important movement—the self-empowerment of thousands of AIDS patients—was quietly going on. The self-empowerment movement had crossover effects on the struggles involving those drugs, but it also had other consequences on its own.

Self-empowerment refers to the idea that people can and should take on action roles for themselves, rather than allowing other people to act on their behalf or make decisions for them. The Burroughs Wellcome protest and the community-based trials of aerolizable pentamidine were carried out by people who agreed with the notion that people infected with, and affected by, HIV should be major actors in the decision-making circles that were determining how and at what price treatment should occur. Self-empowerment with respect to treatment options has taken other forms as well (some of which are discussed in preceding sections of this chapter). Among the more successful endeavors have been bringing in treatments from other countries and "bootlegging" them at home; distributing both types of remedies through underground buyers' clubs; challenging the processes by which new drugs are tested, approved by the FDA, and marketed by pharmaceutical companies; and, when challenges have seemed too time-consuming, conducting tests through community initiatives.

All of the foregoing challenges are parts of the self-empowerment move-ment that occurred on the larger, or systemic, level. Self-empowerment also has to do with how decisions get made on a personal, or individual, level. This kind of self-empowerment is especially important in terms of the relationship between patients and their doctors or other health care providers. People who are not self-empow-ered let their doctors make their decisions for them and don't worry too much about the source of information. People who take a self-empowerment approach, on the other hand, make more decisions for themselves or in partnership with professionals. For instance, they may inform their health care providers of new treatment options; make decisions for themselves about what side effects are worth suffering or whether participation in a clinical trial is a viable option; fire a treat-ment provider who is unsupportive, uninformed, or authoritarian; or go online for a second opinion or further information from other empowered consumers within the AIDS community.

Self-empowerment was not an invention of AIDS activism. It was fostered by women, mainly lesbians, who had been veterans of the earlier women's health movement and had then become active in AIDS work as professionals, volunteers, or activists. The women's health experience that these movement veterans brought encompassed a broad range of tactics, philosophy, and knowledge. One writer de-scribes the women's health movement as a three-part system: health organizations (which publicized problems with the system, educated women about their own bod-ies, and guided consumers to services), new service delivery systems (such as women's clinics and birthing centers), and self-help groups.[38]

The self-help component of this three-part system was particularly valu-able in the women's self-empowerment movement. In the early 1970s, when women were encouraged to examine their own bodies, that self-examination demystified the process of gynecological exams and diagnoses of abnormalities.[39] This self-em-powerment helped women view themselves as experts with regard to their own bodies; this concept was usefully transplanted to the AIDS movement, where HIV-infected people began to regard themselves as experienced and knowledgeable by virtue of having lived with HIV.[40]

Probably the single most direct and dramatic translation from the women's health care movement to the self-empowerment AIDS movement occurred in the unveiling of the Denver Principles. This unveiling occurred early in the self-em-powerment movement; like the demands of the women's health movement before it, it called for action from treatment providers and treatment consumers, as well as general consciousness-raising for the public at-large.

All six of the recommendations made by the Denver Principles for health care professionals directly or indirectly challenge the role of the health care pro-vider as a "detached professional" and suggest ways of connecting with patients on a more personal and equal level. For example, the principles instruct providers to "clearly identify and discuss the theory they favor as to the cause of AIDS, since this bias affects the treatment and advice they give" and "get in touch with their feelings (thoughts, anxieties, hopes, etc.) about AIDS, and not simply deal with AIDS intel-lectually."[41] This approach made several radical assumptions: first, that health care professionals may be wrong (or at least erroneously influenced by their biases); second, that they serve their patients better by attempting to connect with them on a more personal level; and third, that patients are in a position to evaluate the information and ideas of their treatment providers.

These ideas are fortified by the principles enunciated for PWAs, which address the ways they should promote their own rights and responsibilities:

> We recommend that people with AIDS
> 1. Form caucuses to choose their own representatives to deal with the media, to choose their own agenda, and to plan their own strategies.
> 2. Be involved at every level of AIDS decision making and specifically serve on the boards of directors of provider organizations.
> 3. Be included in all AIDS forums with equal credibility as other participants, to share their own experiences and knowledge.
> 4. Substitute low-risk sexual behaviors for those that could endanger themselves or their partners, and we feel that people with AIDS have an ethical responsibility to inform their potential sex partners of their health status.[42]

Together, these four statements from the Denver Principles suggest self-empowerment in all areas of PWAs' daily life, from intimate personal relationships to the highest levels of policymaking.

Although the principles of the PWAs self-empowerment movement were established early on, putting the do-it-yourself approach into practice was tougher. One obvious reason was the huge level of sickness and death among many of the movement's early leaders. Richard Rector, a member of the board of directors of the National Association of PWAs (NAPWA), highlighted a particularly stark example, noting that "in September 1986 the board of directors of NAPWA had 11 members. By the end of October that year, there were only three left. Eight members had died of AIDS during the interval."[43]

A second, perhaps less obvious problem, was that the self-empowerment movement sometimes challenged not only society at large and the federal government but also the very AIDS service and advocacy organizations from which it had sprung. Although most AIDS service organizations were also attempting to practice these self-empowerment principles with their clients, there was an inherent tension between organizations that developed policies and advocated *for their clients* (even when there was significant PWA input) and PWA organizations that performed these functions *for themselves.* At least one author suggests that one of the most important AIDS service organizations in the country, Gay Men's Health Crisis (GMHC) in New York City, was responsible for the demise of the first attempt at PWA organization there, by appropriating or undermining the infant self-empowerment organization's early projects.[44]

Despite these early obstacles, PWA's self-empowerment has found a secure (though not always comfortable) place within the larger AIDS movement. Importantly, although its strongest roots are within the gay community, it has been one of the most important bridges between the gay community and other communities affected by the epidemic. After all, membership in PWA groups is determined, by definition, by HIV infection status rather than sexual orientation or identity within a given social community.

The self-empowerment movement also received a major boost from the advent and spread of the Internet. One of the most important aspects of the self-empowerment concept was that individuals should be allowed to research their medical conditions and make informed decisions regarding their own treatment. In response to this idea and the demand it created, many informational resources have sprung up, seeking to provide HIV-positive people with free, plainly written, and helpful medical information. In some places, a single individual would be the driving force behind a new organization, such as when Martin Delaney began Project Inform in San Francisco in 1985; in others the job would be taken over by a group, such as when ACT UP chapters in several cities set up treatment guides. Still others set up newsletters, such as the twice-monthly *AIDS Treatment News* begun by John James in San Francisco or the *Critical Path* newsletter launched by Kiyoshi Kuromiya in Philadelphia.

These initiatives helped thousands of people in the 1980s in hard-copy form. In the 1990s, however, as self-empowerment activists took to the Internet, their influence spread even further. Like the photocopy technology that preceded it by decades, Internet technology has had a "multiplier effect" by vastly increasing the amount of material that can be made available to people and the potential audience for that material. In earlier times, the availability of medical information was limited to specific places, such as doctor's offices and medical libraries. The advent of treatment newsletters and consumer libraries was an improvement, but a far greater improvement occurred when self-empowerment activists went online. Suddenly, all kinds of treatment information was available to anyone with access to a computer (or access to someone else who could get to a computer).

In the late 1990s, the treatment issues had come full circle, in a sense. Struggles had occurred over all kinds of treatment policy: getting drugs developed and approved, figuring out how to price them and make them available, and deciding who should get to make the final individual treatment decisions. Yet as in all policymaking areas, such decisions are subject to reexamination as circumstances and ideas change.

As time, technology, and self-empowerment progressed, so too did treatment options. To an uncritical observer, it might seem that by the late 1990s, at least the "crisis" phase of the AIDS epidemic was over. Fatalities and serious AIDS-related illnesses were on the decline. Yet simmering beneath the surface of this good news was a new policy struggle. One side of the struggle pointed to the good news—declines in deaths and in progressions from HIV infection to AIDS—but the other pointed instead to bad news: new side effects, new drug-resistant strains of HIV, and exorbitant treatment costs. The culprit that was cited in both cases was a new treatment system: highly active antiretroviral therapy (HAART)—also known as combination therapy or, more simply, "the cocktail."

Most people on both sides of the issue (with the exception of denialists, of course) had to agree that HAART represented a significant advance from the treatment protocols that started in 1987 with the approval of AZT. AZT belongs to a category of drugs called reverse transcriptase inhibitors that work by keeping a virus from replicating at a specific point in the process. The next drug was approved in 1991; didanosine (ddI, Videx) belonged to the same category of drugs. So did the next two approved drugs: zalcitabine (ddC, Hivid) and stavudine (d4T, Zerit) in 1994. A major breakthrough occurred in 1995 when saquinavir mesylate (Invirase) was approved. This new drug worked in a different way to stop HIV; it was the first of a new category of drugs known as protease inhibitors. Several other drugs, including protease inhibitors and reverse transcriptase inhibitors, were also approved in rapid succession, and soon trials were underway to try these drugs in combination with one another.[45] The year 1995 has been called the "year of the demise of monotherapy" (the practice of using one drug at a time as treatment). Researchers quickly went from experimenting with two drugs in combination to the current HAART regimen, which uses two reverse transcriptase inhibitors together with a protease inhibitor.

In June 1997 the federal government in essence gave its stamp of approval to HAART when the Panel on Clinical Practices for the Treatment of HIV Infection within HHS issued a new set of recommendations. The *Washington Post* called the guidelines "a highly unusual effort by the government to redirect treatment of a specific disease."[46] These guidelines were followed by the 1998 release of a "living document" (meaning that it will be subject to further reviews and changes) titled "Guidelines for the Use of Antiretroviral Agents in HIV-Infected Adults and Adolescents."[47] Among the important elements of the 1997 guidelines were the ideas that all PWAs should be on triple therapy; many people with HIV should be on triple therapy as well; and two-drug combinations and monotherapy (except AZT to prevent transmission from pregnant mother to baby) were not recommended.

HHS's statement has several important policy consequences. The statement establishes HAART as the "standard of care" and specifically defines treatment with only two drugs as less than optimal. This statement is important to public- and private-sector policies (as well as those hazy policies that so often come into play in AIDS policymaking) in several ways. One of the most important impacts of these guidelines is on the government itself. The federal government is a major purchaser of drugs for PWAs, through Medicaid (which it splits with the states) and the AIDS Drug Assistance Programs (ADAPs) funded through the Ryan White CARE Act (the subject of chapter 4). In declaring HAART the standard of care, is the federal government in essence is instructing itself to purchase the cocktail for the clients in its care.

The guidelines also have important consequences on the private-sector side. One obvious result is that physicians across the country have been given an important set of instructions regarding the "official" way to treat HIV infection. Similarly, private insurance companies, which often make decisions about what they will and won't cover on the basis of what is considered common practice or the standard of care (as opposed to a treatment or procedure that is still "experimental") have additional reasons to pay for treatment.

Given the precipitous decline in the number of AIDS-related deaths (from an all-time high of approximately 50,000 in 1995 to fewer than 9,000 in 2000),[48] the compelling logic of combination therapy (hit the virus at various points during its replication process), and the HHS guidelines endorsing such treatment, where is the controversy? There is no such thing as a perfect policy solution, and many of the criticisms of HAART therapies arose with the individual drug treatments that preceded it: cost, side effects, accessibility, and who controls the decision process. Two other complications are unique, or at least more problematic to HAART therapy specifically: compliance and drug resistance. Cumulatively, these issues have led many people to question several of the policies being pursued in AIDS drug treatment.

As with most policy issues, increased expenses always bring controversy. There is no denying the fact that HAART, at least as currently priced, is not cheap. Although estimates vary widely, almost all observers put the costs of HAART treatment (medications plus necessary lab tests to monitor them) at approximately $10,000 a year.[49] As AIDS has moved increasingly toward becoming a disease of poor people, the federal government has become increasingly involved in paying the costs of the treatment for AIDS patients. There are two major federally funded programs of health insurance in the United States: Medicaid and Medicare. Medicare is primarily designed to provide health insurance for the nation's elderly population. It also is used to cover disabled persons who qualify for the Social Security Disability Insurance program—a designation that many people with AIDS hold. Even in this aspect, though, it does not enter much into the debate over HAART therapy because Medicare generally does not cover prescription drugs.

Medicaid is different. This joint federal-state program was enacted specifically to provide health insurance coverage to very poor people, and many people with HIV and AIDS fit that description. A General Accounting Office (GAO) report on the funding implications of combination therapy noted that in 1998 Medicaid covered 55 percent of all adult AIDS patients and 90 percent of pediatric AIDS patients.[50]

The GAO report spoke at length about the other major type of government program designed to provide medication for people with HIV and AIDS: ADAPs. These programs were set up to allow the federal government to funnel money through Title II of the Ryan White CARE Act to the states to help them provide funding for prescription drugs for HIV-positive people who are underinsured or uninsured. Because ADAPs are designed to fill the gap in prescription drug coverage, states usually expect ADAP participants to apply for Medicaid first; they then extend ADAP benefits to those who are not Medicaid-eligible but who are still too poor or otherwise unable to get private health insurance. In some places, ADAP also is used to bridge gaps in Medicaid such as limitations on the number of prescriptions a person can get per month.

The cumulative effect of HAART therapy on Medicaid and ADAPs is not hard to guess. Combination therapy is driving costs up—way up. This trend is somewhat less of a problem for Medicaid because Medicaid covers a whole range of medical goods and services. Therefore, if drug costs go up but hospital bills, for example, go down, the overall effect on Medicaid is essentially canceled out. This is not true for ADAPs because these programs exist only to pay for prescription drugs; as more people enroll for more triple therapy, costs will only increase.

The financial strain of providing HAART to an ever-increasing number of people has led to the enactment of several "coping" policies by various states. These policies may stretch ADAP budgets, and they may seriously undermine the original goal of extending optimal treatment to the people who need it most. According to a study conducted by the National Alliance of State and Territorial AIDS Directors cited in the GAO report, in fiscal year 1997 ten states had capped ADAP enrollments; nine states restricted access to the protease inhibitors that are supposed to form an essential element of the cocktail; nine states had waiting lists of people who were eligible but not funded for ADAP enrollment; and seven states had waiting lists of enrolled clients trying to get protease inhibitors. Twelve states also had used money from the Ryan White CARE Act that was supposed to go to other categories of care, such as home health care, to try to make up the shortfalls.

A study being conducted by the AIDS Research Institute of the University of California–San Francisco (UCSF) and scheduled to be released in March 2001 was leaked to AP reporter Laura Meckler in November 2000.[51] The study revealed that, if anything, things had gotten worse. The UCSF study looked at the four states with the highest number of AIDS patients in the United States. According to the study's preliminary findings, Medicaid and ADAPs were failing to deliver appropriate combination therapies to large numbers of their AIDS populations. In Texas, the worst of the four states, almost two-thirds of the state's AIDS patients were not getting the drugs needed for combination therapy. In the other three states (California, Florida, and New York), 40–50 percent of people on Medicaid were getting proper treatment, and two-thirds to three-quarters of these states' ADAP enrollees were receiving the right drugs.[52]

Another serious concern with HAART therapy is that it requires a high level of compliance. The drug combinations work in combination only if there is a sustained level of each drug in the body, which generally means that pills must be taken more than once a day. The regimen is manageable for many HIV-infected people, but for others—such as homeless people, people struggling with drug addiction, and people who don't have much control over their own lives, including prisoners—compliance may be more difficult. Not only must the regimens be followed strictly, but, according to most HAART proponents, they must be followed continuously: Starting means staying for the long haul, although this proposition is coming under increasing scrutiny.

The problems created by the continuous and strict drug regimens of combination therapy have led AIDS advocates (particularly those who are accustomed to questioning conventional wisdom, as the self-empowerment approach encourages) to ask questions of their own. Would it be better to wait before starting to take the AIDS cocktail? What happens if a person starts and has to stop because the side effects are too strong? Is it possible to stop for a limited period of time before going back? All of these questions are being aggressively debated among policymakers; HHS guidelines notwithstanding, there are no hard-and-fast answers.

On one side of the debate are proponents of early and continuous combination therapy. They base their arguments on several claims: HAART helps to prevent viral genetic mutation, thereby decreasing the production of drug-resistant strains; absent aggressive treatment, HIV is free to destroy the immune system in a systematic and relentless way; and there is evidence that early treatment may lead to restoration of some of the body's immune functions.[53]

On the other side, those in favor of later initiation of the cocktail or of interrupted treatment point to the problems of combination therapy: the expense, the side effects, and the related problem of compliance. Combination therapy, like the monotherapies that preceded it, has been associated with numerous side effects. Some, such as gastrointestinal problems, hair loss, and oral warts, are problematic but not life-threatening. Others, such as the lipodystrophy (maldistribution of fat deposits) that create "buffalo humps" and "protease paunches," can cause disfigurement. Still others, such as elevated levels of substances associated with atherosclerosis, lactic acidosis, and hepatic steatosis (a type of liver damage) ultimately may be fatal.

Added to the problem of side effects—and in part a result of it—is the problem of compliance. Studies have shown that most of us are not particularly good at taking our medications as instructed, particularly when it requires multiple daily doses and when we know it might not make us feel well. These conditions are precisely those of most people taking combination therapy, so it is not surprising that researchers have found low levels of compliance in the United States. In an article in the *Journal of the American Medical Association* that argued for "conservative management" (that is, delayed treatment), the authors cited two different studies with disappointing results. In one, only 65 percent of patients on protease inhibitors were found to be adherent to their regimens, even though nonadherence was defined very loosely as failure to pick up two or more monthly prescriptions within a six- to twelve-month period. Similarly, studies of health care workers who thought they might have been exposed to HIV and were given triple therapy as a preventive measure found that a majority reported negative side effects and only 22–56 percent continued their one-month course of medicines.[54]

In a sense, noncompliance is everyone's business. Research shows that failure to take even a few doses of medication increases the chance that a drug-resistant strain of HIV will develop within a patient. This finding has become a potent political argument for proponents of early and continuous therapy; it has also become a major argument embraced by the pharmaceutical industry in the controversies surrounding how to deal with AIDS in Africa (see chapter 6). (As we shall also see, however, treatment activists have some compelling counterarguments to this claim.)

Paradoxically, however, yet another train of thought regarding a treatment option is emerging because of the problems of noncompliance, expense, and side effects. According to this line of thinking, deliberately going off drug therapy for a period of time (not skipping a dose or two or quitting for a couple of days)—dubbed either strategic (or structured) drug interruption (SDI) or strategic treatment interruption (STI)—may not result in the drug resistance but actually may have the opposite effect. That is, it may "reset the clock," in a sense tricking the virus into reverting back to "wild type" as opposed to the mutated forms it may take in the presence of drug therapy. It also gives the patient a psychological and physical break from the constraints and side effects of the therapy. Even proponents of this approach, however, note that viral loads jump way up during drug holidays—often from unde-tectable levels to thousands or even millions of copies of virus per milliliter of plasma.

Although the debate remains open among clinicians, researchers, and AIDS activists, one group in the policy mix has clearly staked out its position: pharmaceu-tical manufacturers of the cocktail. In a community forum on the issue on April 19, 2000, Martin Delaney of Project Inform and Matt Sharp of Survive AIDS (formerly ACT UP Golden Gate) wryly warned the audience not to "expect the drug compa-nies to fund research about stopping medications anytime soon."[55] In their own words, the position becomes still clearer. In two websites offering advice to patients with HIV (www.treathiv.com and www.thepositivesource.com), Glaxo-Wellcome (the expanded successor to Burroughs Wellcome) offers visitors information under the heading "Drug Holidays: One Vacation You Don't Want to Take." The treathiv.com site also offers ten myths about HIV; the first "myth" it debunks is that "taking a drug holiday is good."

In an age of self-empowerment fueled by easy access via computer to a multitude of information, the bottom line on combination therapy is that (currently at least) there is no bottom line. Different policymakers have attempted to create guidelines and rules of thumb, but as the HHS's "living document" exemplifies, they do so knowing that these standards, like the treatment options they suggest, are in a continuous state of flux.

Conclusion

In less than fifteen years we have seen remarkable breakthroughs that addressed the initial demands of many activists: getting drugs into bodies. In the United States, the number of deaths from AIDS has plunged as a result of widespread (though not universal) use of the medications described in this chapter. These drugs have limita-tions, however, and they are not a cure in any sense.

Yet even more fundamentally, the technological solution to HIV and AIDS that the development of these drugs represents only highlights a fundamental limi-tation of all technological solutions. That is, they cannot solve political problems. Even if the drugs that had been developed carried no side effects, many of the policy struggles would still have occurred. There still would have been struggles over how fast the drugs could or should have been developed, which drugs should be tried first, how they should be tested, who should decide how and when to take them, and how much they should cost. All of these decisions are fundamentally political; as such, they have no objectively "correct" answers. Different groups will push for decisions on the basis of their stakes in the game (making a living or need-ing to prolong a life), how much they will gain or lose, and the underlying values that are propelling them to act.

We are unlikely to achieve a nationwide consensus that drugs are a market good like any other and should be treated accordingly, thereby allowing drug com-panies to charge whatever the market will bear, or that health care is a right and government is obligated to provide it, whatever the cost or inconvenience. These two competing positions exemplify a much larger, values-based policy debate in our country. In that larger debate, one side believes that the highest priority should be given to the private market, with its underlying emphasis on individual economic choice. The other side believes in a rights-based approach, with its emphasis on the obligations of the state to provide certain basic goods and services to all its citizens. Barring an extremely unlikely meeting of the minds on this larger values debate within the policy realm, the policy struggle in this area cannot have a permanent political resolution.

CHAPTER 3

Blood Policy in the Age of AIDS

On Saturday, August 19, 2000, a man named Michael Davon died. Dozens of people who had never met him poured out their grief over the Internet as they recounted all he had done for them. He had a degree in computer science from MIT and had worked in the computer industry for more than ten years. Yet he was not mourned as a young and successful dot-com entrepreneur (though he had been a pioneer in the Internet service industry). Rather, he had been professionally sidelined, like thousands of his "blood brothers," through a combination of hemophilia, hepatitis, and HIV. In a letter written to a Vermont senator two years before he died, Michael described what it was like to have to stop working and start dealing with his illness full-time:

> I put off stopping work because of fear and uncertainty about my income and health care. (Would I be forced to become indigent under the weight of the $100,000 or more it cost for my clotting factor, and the $10,000 or more for AIDS drugs, and then there were all those tests and doctor visits and hospitalizations.) Eventually, it was clear to me that I needed to stop and just try and sleep, otherwise I was going to die soon.
>
> My doctor filled out my disability forms and under the "Prognosis" heading wrote "ultimately fatal." Reading this was a bit unsettling.[1]

Yet despite being, as he described with typical understatement, "unsettled," Michael never dealt with his situation passively. Convinced that neither the National Hemophilia Foundation nor the U.S. government had done all they could to prevent his infection with HIV and hepatitis, he helped launch a new organization, the Committee of Ten Thousand, and became one of its longest-serving board members. Later, the hemophilia community went through a difficult and extended attempt to bring a class action suit against the four manufacturers of blood clotting products that Michael and other hemophiliacs required, which resulted in an out-of-court settlement. Believing that justice would require more than the settlement offered, Michael became an "opt-out," preferring to continue to pursue an individual course of action (which never reached fruition in his lifetime). Later still, the hemophilia community demanded that the government take responsibility for its failure to safeguard the blood products it had approved through the Ricky Ray Hemophilia Relief Fund Act. Again, Michael did his part, actively lobbying Congress through letters such as the one excerpted above, which was written from a hospital bed. (As with the lawsuit, Michael never saw a reward in his lifetime for the work he had done.)

It was for none of these reasons, however, that Michael was so widely eulogized, often by people who had never seen his face, when he died. Michael's greatest gift to the hemophilia community was the access he gave community members to each other, through the Internet. In the years before he died, Michael became an Internet philanthropist of sorts, offering free hosting to a w de variety of e-mail lists for communities struggling with various illnesses, includin $ HIV-positive gay men, HIV-positive Spanish-speakers, people with little-known conditions such as Factor V Leiden disease, and, of course, hemophilia. Through the use of the list, the hemophilia community was able to forge a stronger sense of community and a greater level of political power than it had before.

Noting Michael's important contributions to the hemophilia community and, by extension, the politics of blood policy only raises the question of why, however. Why did Michael and thousands like him become infected with HIV? Was it unavoidable? Have policies been corrected to prevent future tragedies? To attempt to answer these questions, we must begin by examining the subject of regulation.

Blood Policy Regulation

In struggles over the creation of policy, the government often has to decide who will be given certain resources and who will lose out. Sometimes, however, the government is called upon to create policies not to distribute something people want but to protect people from something they don't want. In such cases, the government usually is asked to force private individuals or organizations to comply with certain rules. This practice is known as regulation.

Although it's difficult to be opposed to a safer, more protected world in the abstract, government attempts to ensure such a world through regulation almost always create controversy. Who should bear the cost of regulation? How strong should the rules be? When is a danger important enough to demonstrate the need for regulation? Should regulations be enacted if something bad *might* happen or only when we are sure that something bad already has happened? If something bad does happen, who should we hold responsible? These questions, along with many related ones, have been a part of the difficult and controversial creation of the AIDS-related policies that are the subject of this chapter: AIDS and the blood supply.

Unlike many communicable diseases, AIDS is not easily transmitted. There are only a small number of ways that HIV can move from one person to another, and all of them involve some form of physical contact. Yet although there are a very limited number of ways that transmission can occur, one of these—via blood-to-blood contact—is remarkably effective. Hence, although only a small proportion of people are being transfused with blood or blood products at any given time, if those products are HIV-infected, the chances that the transfusion recipient will be infected are very high. For this reason, several actors and groups have had strong stakes in the policies related to maintaining a safe and sufficient supply of blood and blood products.

Keeping track of the groups and issues involved in this policy area can be like reading a play with a very large cast. At first it's hard to keep all the actors straight, but it gets easier when the story unfolds. Before discussing the policy process and how it evolved around the issue of HIV in the blood supply, we must delve into some background information. It is important to know something about the interests of the main actors. It also is useful to understand a bit about how the country's blood policies operated prior to the onset of AIDS in the United States.

There are three categories of groups with strong interests in the development of blood policy: those with a financial stake in the provision of blood and blood products (the blood industry), those whose health depends on the availability of safe blood and blood products (consumers), and those whose job it is to reconcile these two sometimes-competing interests (government regulators). The first group, the blood industry, consists of for-profit and nonprofit private organizations, including the American National Red Cross (ANRC), numerous community blood banks, plasma collection centers, and pharmaceutical companies that manufacture blood products from whole blood or plasma. All of these organizations are engaged in some combination of activities involving the collection, distribution, and processing of blood or blood products. There are three main organizations in the nonprofit sector of the blood industry: the ANRC; the American Association of Blood Banks (AABB), which formed in 1947 as a way to allow local independent blood banks to confederate and compete with the ANRC; and the Council of Community Blood Centers (CCBC), which split from the AABB in 1962. All three of these organizations are involved in collecting, storing, and distributing donated (that is, uncompensated) blood.

Whereas the nonprofit sector deals primarily with whole blood given by unpaid donors, the for-profit sector is involved mainly with plasma and plasma-derived products. There are two main components to the for-profit part of the industry: plasma collection centers and pharmaceutical corporations that manufacture plasma-derived products. Plasma is collected at plasma collection centers through a process called plasmapheresis, whereby blood is taken from the donor and separated into components. The red blood cells and platelets are transfused back into the donor, and the plasma is retained. Relative to whole blood donation, plasmapheresis is a long and uncomfortable process, although a donor can do it safely much more often than with whole blood donations. Unlike whole blood donors, plasma donors are paid a small amount for each donation (eight to twenty-five dollars is typical), and plasma donors tend to be poor people, often with a need for quick money. The plasma that is kept ("source plasma") usually is further processed through fractionation into components known as blood products.

Four companies ("fractionators") control the fractionation part of the plasma industry and manufacture blood products: Armour Pharmaceutical Company, Hyland Therapeutics, Cutter Laboratories, and Alpha Therapeutics. These companies are owned by larger pharmaceutical firms: Armour is a subsidiary of the French company Rhone-Poulenc; Hyland is a subsidiary of Baxter-Travenol; Cutter belongs to A.G. Bayer; and Alpha Therapeutics is owned by the Green Cross Corporation of Japan. One of the most important blood products produced by these four companies is a protein known as antihemophilia factor (AHF), Factor VIII or IX, or sometimes simply "factor." There is a high demand for factor among people with hemophilia because people with this disease lack a protein (usually either Factor VIII or IX) that is necessary during the series of chemical reactions that occur during blood clotting. Before factor was isolated, hemophiliacs were treated with a substance called "cryoprecipitate" that was a mix of proteins, including factor. Before cryoprecipitate was discovered (in the 1960s), hemophiliacs usually were treated (not very effectively) with ice packs or transfusions of whole blood or plasma.

To keep production costs down, fractionators pooled thousands of units of source plasma in the fractionation process. The less sophisticated cryoprecipitate, on the other hand, was produced from much smaller pools. Another cost-cutting measure involved the source of the plasma: plasma collection centers and the fractionators were able to pay plasma donors in U.S. prisons and in poorer countries such as Mexico, Belize, Nicaragua, South Africa, and Haiti a small portion of what they paid in the United States. Hence, plasma collection centers operated among these populations as demand for blood products increased in the 1970s.[2]

By the 1970s, a full-scale "blood industry" was in place. Management of the product had been roughly divided (with some occasional overlap) between nonprofit blood banks that handled whole blood collected from unpaid donors and for-profit plasma collection centers and pharmaceutical companies that collected plasma from paid donors and processed it into components used to treat a variety of medical conditions. The nonprofit end of the industry has a set of internal rules, or standards, established primarily by the AABB through its voluntary accreditation system, which it set up in 1958 for its member organizations.[3]

Both the nonprofit and for-profit sides of the industry are politically represented in Washington, D.C. On the nonprofit side, each of the three major blood banking organizations—the ANRC, the AABB, and the CCBC—maintains representation in decision-making circles relating to blood policy. During the 1980s, one such decision-making group in which the blood industry was (and remains) well-represented, the Blood Products Advisory Committee (BPAC) of the FDA, was particularly crucial in determining how the government would respond to the threat of a new virus in the blood supply. The plasma centers and fractionators of the for-profit sector have their own trade association—the American Blood Resource Association (ABRA), founded in 1971—to represent their interests, and this group also is well-connected to government administrators working with blood policy. The four fractionators also had a second group to articulate their interests: the Pharmaceutical Manufacturers Association.

By the time decisions were being made about HIV infection in the blood supply, the blood industry had well-developed clout in government policymaking. The consumer sector did not, however, for several reasons. First, the largest group affected by blood policy—people who receive blood transfusions—is not an organized group at all. For most of us, blood transfusions are not a central concern in our daily lives. The knowledge that a blood transfusion, if we need it, is safe and accessible constitutes what social scientists refer to as a *diffuse* (as opposed to *concentrated*) benefit. As with most diffuse benefits, few people find themselves strongly motivated to bring together a group of people dedicated to ensuring a benefit that doesn't affect them deeply and immediately.

Prior to the AIDS epidemic, however, there was one major group that constituted an important exception to this rule: people with bleeding disorders, especially hemophilia. For members of this group, access to the new blood products (cryoprecipitate and, better yet, factor) provided by the blood industry was no take-it-or-leave-it benefit. Such access was a genuine *concentrated* benefit from a political science perspective, and just as scholars of interest group organizing would predict, an interest group was developed to represent these consumers: the National Hemophilia Foundation (NHF).

Here, too, however, representation was nowhere near as straightforward as it was for the blood industry. The most important goal of the NHF, from a consumer perspective, was to guarantee affordable access to medical treatment and products that were needed to deal with the complications of bleeding disorders. Although the discovery of factor was a momentous development for the hemophilia community, it presented an additional challenge: cost. Factor enormously simplified the treatment of bleeding episodes and, in some cases, could even be infused preventively to keep bleeding from occurring. The drawback was the expense. Hemophilia and several other bleeding disorders, such as von Willebrand disease, are genetically determined. Not only are the products used to treat them expensive; the disorders themselves are considered "preexisting conditions." This classification made it difficult, if not impossible, for people with these disorders to acquire health insurance in the 1970s, before laws were passed making it more difficult to discriminate against those with preexisting conditions.

In recognition of this and other cost problems, the NHF led a successful effort to get federal funding for comprehensive hemophilia treatment centers (HTCs). This quest for government aid culminated in the July 1975 passage of Public Law 94-63, which included funding for twenty-six centers.[4] Once the HTCs had been established and AHF was widely available, the hemophilia community entered what would later be recalled nostalgically as its "golden age."

There was a hidden danger to this new arrangement, however. During this period the interests of physicians, the blood industry, and people with hemophilia all appeared to converge. Although the NHF was created to serve people with bleeding disorders, it actually served three constituencies: consumers, their health providers (usually working through the HTCs), and the providers' suppliers. The common interest was factor itself: It helped people with hemophilia avoid the pain and disabling consequences of uncontrolled bleeds, it allowed treatment professionals to prosper as successful clinicians, and it made the blood industry a lot of money.

The situation got worse in the late 1970s, when the NHF slipped into "technical bankruptcy."[5] The NHF's executive director was dismissed in February 1979; the acting executive director who followed quit after only a few months, and the executive director who followed him was terminated by the end of the year. In the meantime, the activities of the organization were kept afloat in large part by money donated by the fractionators to the NHF's medical codirectors for programs, "to produce educational publications for both professional and lay audiences and also to support meetings for newly formed professional committees."[6]

Thus, in contrast to the blood industry, advocacy for consumers was either nonexistent (for transfusion recipients) or compromised (for those with bleeding disorders). The only organization charged to speak in Washington policymaking circles about blood policy was the NHF, but that organization had more than one master. On one hand, it was supposed to advocate for an adequate, safe, and afford-able supply of blood and blood products. On the other hand, it was accepting money from the very companies whose positions on these same issues often were radically different from the NHF's.

The third major set of actors was the government agencies charged to regu-late and research blood disorders and blood policy. Although several agencies had responsibilities in these areas, in the crucial area of blood safety, one group—the FDA—had a role that far eclipsed the others, at least on paper. Other government agencies that have had a role in research or regulation regarding hemophilia products included NIH—particularly the National Heart, Lung and Blood Institute (NHLBI), whose job is to research hemophilia, and the NIAID, whose job is to research AIDS. In addition, the CDC, whose job is to track the incidence and spread of diseases and to help prevent that spread, had a crucial role in the debates over how to slow the spread of HIV in the blood supply. Prior to the AIDS epidemic, however, the CDC did not have direct links to the groups who determined most blood policy, and this lack of connection had serious consequences when the agency entered the debate.

Since 1972, the agency with the most direct role in regulating blood and blood products has been the FDA. Within the FDA, control over blood and blood product regulation has shifted around a bit. First (in 1972) it fell to the Bureau of Biologics, then (in 1982) to the Center for Drugs and Biologics, and finally (in 1988) to the Center for Biologics and Review. In 1993 this last group was renamed the Center for Biologics Evaluation and Research (CBER), and regulation of blood and blood products is centered at the CBER today.[7]

While regulatory control within the FDA was being shuffled around dur-ing the 1980s, a key group for regulatory policy was much more stable. This group was the BPAC. Although the FDA technically is in charge of creating and enforcing regulations regarding the safety of various products, it relies heavily on outside ad-visory committees for advice on technical issues and how a proposed decision or regulation might affect the industry being regulated. In this respect, the BPAC was typical of other advisory committees. During the early 1980s the blood industry was well represented on the BPAC, but consumers were not. This pattern in large part reflected the prevailing notion at the time that technical issues of blood policy would be "over the heads" of consumers and were best left to the "experts."

Denial and Disaster: Early Reactions to the Blood Supply Threat

In 1982 a new development exposed the flaws of the interdependent network that created blood policy in the United States. That new development was the discovery of a new disease among people with hemophilia. On July 6, 1982, Dr. Bruce Evatt of the CDC sent a letter to Dr. Louis Aledort, medical codirector of the NHF, notifying him of the first three cases of immunosuppression in hemophiliacs. He specifically noted that the causal agent appeared to be transmitted in the same ways as the hepatitis virus. Thus, Evatt warned, "Hemophiliacs would be prime candidates to develop this syndrome." This letter was followed on July 9 with a mass mailing to state and territo-rial health officers to inform them of this news as well.

Then, on July 27, 1982, an emergency meeting of the Public Health Services Committee was called. Invitees included representatives of the CDC, FDA, NIH, NHF (including Dr. Aledort), ANRC, AABB, CCBC, the pharmaceutical industry, and the gay community. Although this meeting would be notable for formally naming the new disease acquired immune deficiency syndrome, or AIDS, it later also became notable for what it did not do. Despite the exhortations of CDC representatives, the attendees decided that the best course of action would be to study the issue further and continue to monitor the situation. Specifically, they did *not* recommend that the use of factor or other blood products should be limited in any way or that donor blood or plasma be screened or tested in any way.[8]

Ten days prior to this meeting, the NHF had sent out an alert in its *Hemophilia Newsnotes,* telling its readership that "the *risk* of contracting this immunosuppressive agent is *minimal* and CDC is not recommending any change in blood product use" (emphasis in original). To emphasize the point, it went so far as to add a second message at the bottom of the sheet (double spaced, in capital letters) that read, "Important: Remember, CDC is not advising a change in treatment at this time. If there are any questions, contact your physician or hemophilia treatment center."[9] Similar *Newsnotes* went out until at least 1984, when—even as it reported a recall for an HIV-contaminated lot of clotting factor—the NHF issued its Medical Bulletin #10/Chapter Advisory #13, titled "NHF Reaffirms Position that Product Withdrawal Should Not Change Use of Clotting Factor." After discussing the withdrawal and NHF policy regarding recalls, the newsletter emphasized (again in bold-faced capital letters):

> Most important, despite the concern that may be raised by the recall of plasma products, the NHF reaffirms its recommendation that patients maintain the use of concentrate, or cryoprecipitate as prescribed by their physicians. The life and health of hemophiliacs depends upon the appropriate use of blood products.[10]

The risk of HIV transmission from infected hemophiliacs to their sexual partners was similarly downplayed. After the January 1984 *Annals of Internal Medicine* published an account of HIV transmission from a seventy-year-old hemophiliac to his wife, the NHF responded with two directives—one to its consumer members (Chapter Advisory #14) and one to physicians only (Medical Bulletin #11). The Chapter Advisory noted the reported case but added the (incorrect) reassurance that "in the medical and scientific community there are different points of view on this topic but all agree that *if* sexual partners are at increased risk for AIDS, *this risk is remote*" (emphasis in original).[11]

The Medical Bulletin stressed that "because of the sensitive nature of the material contained in the Bulletin, it is intended for providers only" but warned providers that Chapter Advisory #14 "will likely provide distressing concern" and counseled that "the usual preventive measures should be employed, that is, open discussion such as chapter meetings involving center staff. This provides a forum for ventilation and reassurance."[12] Significantly, no suggestion was made anywhere in the bulletin for counseling regarding safer sex practices.

Yet it was not true that the CDC saw no new risks to hemophiliacs. Following the inconclusive July 1982 meeting, a second meeting with expanded participation was called on January 3, 1983. In this meeting—officially termed the Workgroup to Identify Opportunities for Prevention of Acquired Immune Deficiency Syndrome—the CDC earned the enmity of many of the other participants by arguing that serious measures be taken to protect the blood supply by screening potentially high-risk donors and testing the blood with a "hepatitis core test." The NHF supported screening of donors, but gay rights groups opposed such testing because they felt that it would stigmatize a whole group because of the status of a few members. Dr. Oscar Ratnoff proposed reverting to the use of cryoprecipitate made from pools of ten or fewer donors, rather than factor, but this strategy was opposed by the drug companies and other hemophilia doctors, who argued (wrongly, it turned out) that the results, in terms of transmission of the new syndrome, would be the same.

The core testing idea hinged on the discovery that nearly 90 percent of known AIDS cases in the United States at the time also tested positive for hepatitis B. Although blood banks already routinely screened for a surface hepatitis B antibody that detected recent hepatitis exposure, the CDC was suggesting testing for the presence of the virus core that remained in the body for years. Given the 90 percent correlation, the presence of the core antibody would serve as a "surrogate marker" for the yet-to-be-discovered AIDS virus.[13]

Dr. Bruce Voeller of the gay rights-based group Physicians for Human Rights supported the idea of surrogate testing rather than donor screening, as did Roger Enloe of the National Gay Task Force.[14] The blood industry strongly disagreed. Blood bankers pointed to the cost and the fact that a significant fraction of their donor base would be lost. They also argued that the CDC had yet to prove its argument. In the words of Dr. Aaron Kellner, director of the New York Blood Center, the CDC had "three cases at most, and the evidence in two of these cases is very soft."[15] Dr. Louis Aledort of the NHF also counseled caution, arguing that time would bring more evidence to bear. These statements enraged Dr. Don Francis, a CDC veteran of previous epidemics. Pounding his fist on the table, he demanded that the others in the room tell him how many people had to die before there would be compelling evidence for action.

The aftermath of this meeting was not a pronouncement of government policy but a flurry of activity within the blood industry. The nonprofit end of the blood industry (the ANRC, AABB, and CCBC) held a meeting of its own on January 6 to create a Joint Task Force Against AIDS, and the NHF met with the blood industry for a strategy meeting on January 14. Prior to this strategy meeting, the industry met privately to determine a "consensus strategy."

The three blood banking groups (ANRC, AABB, and CCBC) issued a joint statement on January 13. Noting that the "possibility of blood-borne transmission, still unproven, has been raised," these groups suggested seven specific measures, including educational campaigns for doctors, autologous transfusions, screening of donors for the symptoms of AIDS (e.g., nights sweats and Kaposi's sarcoma), and redirection of recruitment drives away from high-risk groups. Specifically rejected were questioning about a donor's sexual preference ("Direct or indirect questioning about a donor's sexual preference are inappropriate") and surrogate testing ("We do not advise routine implementation of any laboratory screening program for AIDS at this time").[16] Meanwhile, at the NHF/industry summit the NHF began to push for tough screening and surrogate testing, as well as issuance of some precautions about cutting back on the use of factor (although in its publications to the community, the NHF generally continued to advise the use of factor).[17]

In addition to the public meetings and statements being issued, internal memos that were being circulated revealed a specific strategy for dealing with the crisis, at least in the short term. Simply put, that strategy was to shut out the alarmist government agency (the CDC) and take direction from the more accommodating agency (the FDA). A Red Cross internal memo, for instance, reveals a poorly concealed contempt for the CDC's perceived overzealousness:

> Even if the evolving evidence of an epidemic wanes CDC is likely to continue to play up AIDS—it has long been noted that CDC increasingly needs a major epidemic to justify its existence. This is especially true in light of Federal funding cuts and the fact that AIDS probably played some positive role in CDC's successful battle with [the Office of Management and Budget] to fund a new $15,000,000 virology lab. This CDC perspective is also obvious from the general "marketing nature" of the January 4, 1983, Atlanta meeting (e.g., abundant press at a "scientific" meeting, presentation without hard copy, hard selling [surrogate] testing, etc). In short, we can *not* depend on CDC to provide scientific, objective, unbiased leadership on this topic.[18]

An internal memo of Cutter Laboratories is even more straightforward. Summarizing the consensus strategy the blood industry had reached in its meeting prior to the NHF/industry summit, the memo noted plans to "support testing in concept, but defer until a more specific test was available." Regarding the CDC, "we also agreed that the CDC was increasingly involved in areas beyond their expertise, and whenever possible we would try to deflect activity to NIH/FDA."[19]

The deflection of authority to the FDA had the desired effect of less-than-total response to the new threat. On March 24, 1983, the Office of Biologics within the FDA released recommendations to "Establishments Collecting Source Plasma" (the for-profit industry) and "Establishments Collecting Human Blood for Transfusion" (the nonprofit industry). Noting that the steps outlined were consistent with the recommendations made by various members of the blood industry, both sets of guidelines included measures for conducting voluntary self-exclusion by donors, ways of deferring donors by looking for physical symptoms of AIDS, and measures for disposing of blood or plasma that was believed to be contaminated.[20] Significantly, neither direct questioning of sexual or other risk behaviors nor surrogate testing was recommended in either set of directives.

Despite the official recommendations from the FDA, a few maverick blood banks took precautions on their own. Dr. Edward Engleman of Stanford University's hospital blood bank undertook his own testing, using a T4/T8 ratio test that detected a blood cell abnormality that was typical among people carrying the AIDS virus but not yet showing other signs of AIDS. Although the test cost $10 per donation and did not perfectly identify all cases, he felt that it was superior to doing nothing. The blood industry rejected his approach, however, arguing that the case for blood-borne contamination still had not been proven and, further, that the expense was too great.[21] In December 1983 the BPAC of the FDA met to discuss yet again the idea of using surrogate testing. Rather than recommending surrogate testing, the BPAC agreed to an idea from the blood industry to create an industry task force to continue examining the issue.[22] Not surprisingly, this task force issued an interim report three months later concluding that hepatitis B core testing was "not appropriate" for screening donors.[23]

While the blood industry resisted the implementation of testing and screening rules that, it argued, would only cause shortages in the blood supply, there were additional complications related to the products used by people with hemophilia. One controversy revolved around the introduction of a heat treatment process for factor, and a second dilemma arose over the question of recalls of tainted products.

The first issue, heat treatment, had a history before the age of AIDS. Although factor clinically was a great improvement over cryoprecipitate, it was made by pooling the plasma of thousands of donors. These donors, in turn, often were people who desperately needed money, including people with drug addiction problems and prisoners, and were at higher risk demographically for hepatitis than the general population. The resulting factor products were often hepatitis infected; consequently, the vast majority of hemophiliacs who were treated with factor were infected with hepatitis.

Despite widespread hepatitis infection within the hemophilia community, attempts to find procedures to reduce or eliminate viral contamination were half-hearted, at best. Dr. Edward Shanbrom, a pioneering scientist in fractionation, developed a detergent method of killing hepatitis, but, in his own words, "No one expressed interest, not a soul."[24] Several reasons have been offered for the slow activity in this area: Some people believed that a hepatitis B vaccine was very close at hand; because most hemophiliacs were already infected, uncontaminated factor was a moot point; and heat-treated AHF would be more expensive and less effective.[25] In short, "the hemophilia treatment community considered the risk of hepatitis to be an acceptable price to pay for the benefits of AHF concentrate."[26]

Although all of these reasons may have played into the decision by the blood industry not to aggressively pursue heat treatment, a lesser-known factor also may have played a part—and would play an important role in later litigation as well. This other factor was a set of state statutes collectively known as "blood shield laws." Beginning with California in 1955, states passed these laws at the request of doctors, hospitals, and the blood industry, all of whom were concerned about liability issues involved in transmission of hepatitis through blood and blood products. According to these laws, blood was redefined from being a product to being a service. This legal fiction was significant: The difference is that services do not carry the implied warranty and strict liability that products do. Thus, people who received tainted blood or blood products had to prove that there had been actual negligence or misconduct on the part of the supplier, rather than (as with, for example, a tainted medication) simply that the product had been defective. In simple terms, blood shield laws effectively shielded not the consumer of blood or blood products but the suppliers—who, in case after case, walked away victorious when they were brought to court.

Just as manufacturers were not enthusiastic about finding viral inactivation methods for their products, they also were hesitant about instituting product re- calls. The main thrust of their argument in the product recall controversy was that automatic recalls would result in product shortages. This position was promoted at a July 1983 meeting of the BPAC that was called to discuss this very issue. The problem, according to the interest group representing the fractionators, the Phar- maceutical Manufacturers Association, was that a single donor could be represented in as many as fifty plasma pools in a year. If that person were found to have AIDS and all clotting concentrate that had been in the same pool with his donations were withdrawn, there could be "serious disruption of supply."[27] Acting on these argu- ments of the blood industry, the BPAC decided to support a policy of viewing the recall of lots of factor as "discrete events." This decision meant that each lot to which a person who was known to have AIDS had donated would be treated on a case-by-case basis, considering three factors: how reliable the diagnosis of AIDS in the donor was, when the donor showed symptoms in relation to when he or she had donated, and the effect that withdrawal would have on the supply of factor.[28] Inter- estingly, the issue of recalls apparently was taken up by the BPAC in the first place only because representatives of the NHF had brought a proposal to the table. Thus, the interests of consumers with hemophilia were at least nominally represented, although the policy affecting them ultimately was decided in favor of the interests of the blood industry. The other large group of consumers—recipients of blood transfusions and non-factor blood products—had no representation, and the issue of recalls for whole blood and plasma was never even discussed.[29]

Although disruption of supply may have been a real concern, clearly so was the profit motive. One piece of evidence that demonstrated the sacrifice of safety to profits came with the unearthing of a confidential internal memo of Cutter Labora- tories. The March 20, 1986, memo, which was written after the institution of anti- body testing and heat treatment, lists the "issue" as requests from various sources to have material that has been screened for HIV. The "decisions" in response to this issue include putting "unscreened material into finished inventory as soon as pos- sible," keeping to a general rule of *not* distinguishing between screened and unscreened lots, and telling the people in distribution to "move existing unscreened finished good inventory before we move screened material."[30]

Eventually the blood industry did find ways to virally inactivate AHF. In 1983 Baxter's Hyland Division became the first company to receive an American patent for heat treatment; and by 1984 all four fractionators had FDA approval and were heat-treating at least some of their product for hepatitis.[31] At first the NHF was hesitant to recommend the new heat-treated product. In October 1984, how- ever, after the AIDS virus had been identified and the labs of the CDC and one of the fractionators (Cutter) had shown that it was killed by heat treatment, the NHF suggested that doctors "strongly consider" using heat-treated products.[32]

Even the introduction of heat-treated factor did not put an end, however, to the threat of receiving HIV-contaminated blood products. Although heat treatment had become standard procedure by 1985, the FDA waited until 1989 to require that manufacturers recall and destroy all untreated units. Several reasons have been offered for this hesitancy on the part of the FDA. At least initially, the FDA did not have actual proof that the heat-treated concentrates actually were safer. There also was some concern that heat treatment might cause other problems, such as reactions to the factor. Other blood bankers and factor producers argued that many patients were already presumed to be virally infected at this point anyway, and heat-treated factor was more expensive. For these reasons, there also was resistance to prescribing it on the part of hemophilia doctors,[33] and the FDA may have been reluctant to push these doctors. In a retrospective study of the decisions made during this period, the Committee to Study HIV Transmission Through Blood and Blood Products concluded, however, that many of these reasons were not well-founded themselves and that "there seems to be no reason to believe that the transition from untreated to treated AHF concentrate could not have been accomplished faster with active agency leadership."[34]

Two important events related to blood safety occurred in the mid-1980s. The first was the introduction of heat-treated factor, which was initially licensed in 1983 and was prescribed routinely by 1985. Heat treatment was never an option, however, for whole blood because it destroyed red blood cells. The important breakthrough for this side of the blood industry came with the introduction of an actual HIV antibody test, which occurred in April 1985—approximately one year after the announcement of the discovery of HIV as the virus that causes AIDS. Initial resistance came from gay rights groups, which feared (accurately, in many cases) that the antibody test would become a tool for discriminating against HIV-positive people by insurers, employers, and others, and from blood bankers who questioned whether they were obligated to conduct the notifications that a testing system would require and objected to the loss of blood that would occur because of false positive results.[35] Despite these objections, four months after testing at the blood banks began a conference held by NIH and the FDA concluded that testing was a success, and such tests became institutionalized as a part of the blood donation process.[36]

The early and mid-1980s were a time in which the blood industry, advocacy groups, and government agencies struggled over the question of how to prevent transmission of HIV through blood and blood products. Once screening, testing, and heat treatment (later supplemented with the development of recombinant products that did not require human plasma) were selected as the main policy responses to this problem, however, another question rose to the fore: Who was responsible for the unfortunate people who had been infected with HIV *before* these policies were implemented?

What Does Justice Look Like?

Although no one knows exactly how many people in the United States were infected with HIV via blood and blood products, we do know that the number is in the thousands. According to an early estimate by the CDC, 9,465 (63 percent) of the estimated 15,500 hemophiliacs in the United States were believed to have been infected in this way.[37] By December 1998 the CDC had reported a total of 5,603 cases of AIDS related to hemophilia or clotting disorders;[38] this figure is a count of the number of reported AIDS cases, however, not the number of people with HIV infection. An even larger number—approximately twice as many people, in fact—were infected through infected blood transfusions, according to CDC estimates.[39]

Despite these infection levels, however, neither people with hemophilia nor those with transfusion-related HIV initially organized to seek redress for their conditions. The reasons for inactivity among these two groups are very different. In the case of transfusion-related AIDS, the simplest reason for the lack of initial response was that there is no such thing as a "transfusion community." People who share the fact that they have been given a blood transfusion have little else in common. Transfusions are "diffuse benefits," and people rarely organize to obtain such diffuse benefits. Thus, when a group of very different people leading very different lives wound up with HIV infections from their blood transfusions, there was no existing group, or even important shared experience, to pull them together, at least initially.

The situation among hemophiliacs was very different. Although hemophilia is a genetic condition, and hemophiliacs therefore are widely geographically dispersed, earlier experiences had forged a sense of community among people with hemophilia. They had a shared experience of dealing with a lifelong chronic condition, and most of them had lived through the "bad old days" before cryoprecipitate and factor had made treatment much easier. Furthermore, they were connected through the NHF, which had local chapters around the country; through publications, meetings, and sometimes even summer camps sponsored by the NHF (and often funded by the fractionators); and through regional HTCs. The impediment to organization among hemophiliacs was not a lack of community, rather a community ethic that emphasized privacy over activism.

Although the late 1980s was a period of major activism by others infected with and affected by HIV, the hemophilia community was not a part of this wave of activism. It is true that several hemophiliacs—especially school-aged hemophiliacs—found themselves in the position of being the epidemic's new "poster children." In fact, in a study that examined all AIDS news stories appearing on the three major broadcast television networks from January 1, 1981, through April 1, 1987, analysts found a marked propensity to devote a disproportionate amount of news coverage to hemophiliacs and people who contracted HIV through blood transfusions, especially children, and to portray these cases in a way that stressed their status as innocent victims.[40]

This media attention often was organizationally counterproductive, however. It often emphasized exactly the dangers of going public with an HIV-positive status. Seeing Ryan White being spurned by his school when he attempted to attend class in 1985 or watching stories of the Ray brothers being banned from their Florida school in 1987 and having their house burned down only heightened the fears of people who still had not disclosed their status to their communities. In a 1994 editorial in the activist magazine *The Common Factor,* Greg Haas argued that the NHF "chose to shepherd the fears of the community instead of confronting the reality."[41]

Yet others would argue retrospectively that activists such as Haas were engaged in revisionist history: Glenn Pierce, chair of the NHF's AIDS task force, recalls that he developed a white paper about AIDS among people with hemophilia, only to have its distribution voted down by local chapters and the NHF board of directors:

> The chapters just got up in arms and said, "You can't do this, we have people living in this community. If they're exposed, their house could be destroyed, this will happen, they'll be kicked out of school." So this White Paper never saw the light of day. It's important to point out, because that was really the mentality of our grassroots community. When the behavior of the NHF is criticized today, in retrospect, NHF's behavior as an organization was consistent with what our constituents wanted. It's revisionist history, and the people who are the loudest critics of what the organization was doing in the 1980s were as deep in the closet as you can get. In fact, in many cases their chapters didn't even know about them.[42]

Another impediment to activism derived from the fact that there were important divisions between the hemophilia and gay communities, and the gay community was the basis for most early AIDS activism. In addition to the disagreements that had arisen in earlier struggles over whether to screen out gay men as blood and plasma donors, there was the problem created by the media coverage of the hemophilia community. The characterization of hemophiliacs as "innocent victims" tended to juxtapose them against other people with AIDS, particularly those who had acquired HIV through gay sex. The strong implication was that if a person with HIV was not "innocent" (that is, had not acquired the virus through a transfusion), he or she therefore must somehow be "guilty."

All of these factors had the combined effect of stalling activism within the hemophilia community; when it did occur, it began with uncoordinated individual efforts. One of the earliest such efforts was an attempt at internal reform of the NHF in 1988. This effort was undertaken by Dana Kuhn, a mild hemophiliac who had been infected with HIV from a single infusion of factor in 1983. Kuhn had joined the NHF board of directors and from this position helped to launch the Man's Advocacy Network of NHF (MANN). MANN was initiated to help alleviate the perceived power imbalance that was working against NHF's consumer constituency, but it was a reformist, not radical, organization. It operated with the presumption that reform from within was an optimal goal. In 1993 the limits of such reform were stretched too far, however, in the view of the NHF board of directors. At a May meeting of the board, Kuhn suggested, with the backing of MANN, that an investigational committee be set up to research allegations about Executive Director Allan Brownstein (who later resigned under pressure from MANN and other outside groups). Rather than granting the request, the board passed a vote of confidence in Brownstein, and Kuhn resigned.

While Kuhn was working at reform from within, others had decided to take a more radical route outside of NHF. These groups had begun to bridge the gap between the hemophilia and gay communities, and they showed clear signs of the influence of radical activist groups such as ACT UP. From their slogans ("Action = Life," "No More Business as Usual," "Cry Bloody Murder") to their tactics (demonstrations, lawsuits, demands for investigations) to their targets (the blood industry, the FDA, and even the NHF itself), these groups clearly were different from those that had been represented by the NHF in the past.

Geographically, the new activists were concentrated along the coasts of the country, with one hot spot of development around Boston and the other in northern California. The Boston organization, the Committee of Ten Thousand (COTT—named after the estimated 10,000 hemophiliacs who had become infected with HIV), began in 1989 as a peer-led support group.[43] Its founder, however—Jonathan Wadleigh, who also attended meetings of ACT UP Boston and had a background of civil rights activism—quickly moved to infuse the organization with a more political and activist focus. With several fellow hemophiliacs, including Greg Haas, who was from a family that had been active in the NHF, and Tom Fahey, who brought his expertise as a counselor, Wadleigh launched COTT's publication, *The Common Factor*, in April, 1991.[44] This publication was dedicated to covering treatment options, issues of HIV and sexuality, and "the science, business and politics of HIV and hemophilia."

Meanwhile, in northern California the Hemophilia/HIV (H/HIV) Peer Association was founded in 1991 by political scientist-turned-journalist Michael Rosenberg. For Rosenberg, the issue was clear: Hemophiliacs had been betrayed by the blood industry, the NHF, and especially the doctors who had treated them.

In addition to the formation of these two groups, the early 1990s saw the transformation of some existing ones. Several individual state and regional chapters of the NHF defected from the national organization, including the Hemophilia Associations of Acadiana and New Jersey and Hemophilia Northwest. In May 1993 these new groups banded together into a new national consortium, the Hemophilia Federation of America. Among the rules decided upon at its founding were stipulations that there be no funding by the makers of factor or other blood products and that any person who financially benefited from the sale or production of blood products would not be allowed to serve in a voting capacity on the federation's Coordinating Council.[45] The spirit of the new federation was exemplified by its first enunciated goal: "to empower its constituents in order to achieve an equitable relationship with medical professionals and with the pharmaceutical industry."[46]

These three new organizations—particularly COTT and the H/HIV Peer Association—were much more radical in orientation than the NHF. COTT was strengthened when California hemophilia activists Corey Dubin and Leo Murphy began a second chapter, COTT West, in 1993. The publications put out by the Peer Association and COTT—*Action Now* and *The Common Factor*, respectively—were explicitly political and made strong claims about problems with the nation's blood system and the need for redress in the hemophilia community. Equally important, the new activist organizations explicitly embraced other groups within AIDS activism, as well as other rights-based movements. Like these groups, they became willing to openly question, demonstrate against, and even take legal action against the former sacred cows of their world: HTCs, government officials, suppliers of blood products, and the NHF.

Equally important for the movement toward a more activist position was these groups' decision to dissociate themselves from the sympathetic but constricting status of "innocent victim" bestowed on them first by the media and later by the general public. Regarding the victim concept as disempowering and unnecessarily divisive within the larger AIDS community with which they were striving to ally themselves, these groups attempted to replace it with a greater ethos of solidarity. They found common cause with other AIDS activists against industries that were profiting from sickness, government officials who were too timid to act, and a general public that was misinformed about diseases such as hemophilia and AIDS. In an editorial in *The Common Factor*, Greg Haas gave voice to these ideas:

> Persons with hemophilia are but one underserved community. Women, inner city and rural populations, persons of color, incarcerated people and others all are confronted with similar barriers to clinical trials and influence within the research system. We cannot stand apart, pretending our mode of transmission makes us innocent victims.
>
> As long as we consider ourselves victims we cannot act. There is no innocence. There is no guilt. There is infection. There is death. We must add our voices to the struggles of all of the communities affected by this damn virus.[47]

Despite these new alliances with the larger AIDS community, the activist hemophilia community had a separate agenda that it began to pursue. Although Greg Haas and others wrote eloquently about avoiding the blame game, those sentiments did not extend to government and the blood industry. As more and more information became available about the foot-dragging that the blood banks and fractionators had engaged in and the FDA had allowed, the sadness within the hemophilia community turned to anger and a deep desire for accountability. This desire crystalized into several important goals: official government investigations into what went wrong and who was at fault; compensation from the fractionators and the federal government; and representation in decision-making circles to mitigate the chance of future disasters. (Although most of these projects were initiated in the early 1990s and therefore overlapped chronologically, I examine them separately in this discussion.)

During the early 1990s the hemophilia community—beginning with the H/HIV Peer Association's Michael Rosenberg—began to call on Congress to conduct an official investigation. In response to these calls, senators Edward Kennedy (D-Mass.) and Robert Graham (D-Fla.) and Representative Porter Goss (R-Fla.) sent a letter to HHS Secretary Donna Shalala in April 1993, asking her to open an investigation. She passed the charge to the Institute of Medicine (IOM), which formed a special committee of fourteen experts (notably, however, *not* people who had been outspoken on the issues at hand) known as the Committee to Study HIV Transmission Through Blood and Blood Products.

The hemophilia community initially was disappointed at the appointment for several reasons: the committee was not an actual congressional committee; it would not have the same media-grabbing capacity that a congressional committee might; it would not have subpoena power; and it was specifically not to attribute blame but only to provide guidance for better practices in the future.[48] Nevertheless, the committee was an important beginning, and the hemophilia community put its opportunities to good use. Activist Dana Kuhn, with a handful of others, had compiled an impressive array of documents that were bound together and collectively entitled "The Trail of AIDS in the Hemophilia Community." This collection included internal memos and other communications from within the blood industry, the NHF, and government agencies within the FDA, and Kuhn happily handed these documents over to the new committee. The committee itself held several meetings during its year-long investigation, including a public hearing where fifty-nine speakers testified and another fifty provided written statements.

The community's access to the committee was clearly evident in the results, which were issued in a book-length report on July 13, 1995. The committee's publication, *HIV and the Blood Supply: An Analysis of Crisis Decisionmaking*, claims that it "does not seek to determine liability or affix blame for any individual or collective decisions regarding HIV transmission through blood or blood products"[49] yet it is almost impossible not to read some fault-finding into the committee's conclusions.

Like the activist hemophiliacs who had called for the investigation, the IOM committee found that the very organization that was supposed to advocate for the hemophilia community, the NHF, had some serious problems. The NHF's interdependence with the fractionators, the committee found, had led to NHF recommendations that "reflected conflicts of interest, were not adequately objective, and seriously compromised NHF's credibility."[50] In addition, the communication style of the NHF and its Medical and Scientific Advisory Committee (MASAC) was found to be paternalistic and insufficient in meeting the informational needs of its constituency.[51]

The committee found plenty of problems with the FDA and the blood industry as well. The FDA, as the agency that is supposed to oversee the blood industry and overrule potentially bad industry decisions, took the most heat. Among other findings, the committee found that the blood industry could have developed heat treatment processes before 1980, thereby preventing many of the AIDS cases among hemophiliacs that ultimately developed.[52] It also found that the FDA took too much advice from the BPAC and that the BPAC was too controlled by the commercial interests that were represented on it.[53] Finally, in the issue of blood collection, the IOM committee found that the blood banks and the FDA had unreasonably dragged their feet; in instance after instance, they "consistently chose the least aggressive option that was justifiable."[54]

Although the report made recommendations for correcting the wrongs it found, it did not carry the force of law, and HHS Secretary Shalala had to decide how to implement it. The report itself was partial vindication for some activists in the community, but to many others it was a poor substitute for the justice they sought. For them it was a simple matter: Those responsible, in government and in private corporations, must pay. The first attempts to gain this type of justice were individual: People who had used infected factor and their survivors began to bring lawsuits against the fractionators who had produced the factor. What they quickly found, however—as did those who got HIV from tainted blood transfusions—is that their suits were routinely thrown out, sometimes without even being heard.

The biggest problem was the blood shield laws. By defining blood and blood products as "services" rather than "products," they eliminated the strict liability and implied warranty that products carry. If blood products carried such strict liability and implied warranty, a person who contracted HIV would need to show merely that the HIV was contracted through the contaminated product. Without these two conditions, however, the person must also show that the contamination occurred because the entity that manufactured the product did it in a negligent way—that is, in a way that was more negligent than what the rest of the industry was doing. As we have seen, however, the entire blood industry had been unified in its refusal to screen blood and plasma, and none of the fractionators had heat treated factor in the early 1980s. Given these conditions, how was a single plaintiff to show that an individual blood bank or fractionator was any more negligent than any other? Not surprisingly, the vast majority of such cases ended in victory for the defendant.

For the hemophilia community, an additional factor added insult to injury: the position of the NHF and many hemophilia doctors regarding these suits. The NHF had argued against lawsuits on several grounds, including privacy concerns and, later, that a more collaborative approach embodied by its Special Assistance Council (SAC), using voluntary contributions from industry, would better serve the community. These arguments were roundly rejected by politicized hemophilia activists.

To activist Michael Rosenberg, what was even worse was the behavior of hemophilia doctors who testified on behalf of the fractionators in trials. Several important hemophilia doctors who testified for fractionators in trials about the "state of knowledge" regarding AIDS in the early 1980s were put on "shame lists" by the H/HIV Peer Association, and the head of the NHF's MASAC, Dr. Louis Aledort, was labeled the "Mengele" of the "hemophilia holocaust."[55]

Not surprisingly, during the early 1990s the NHF's annual conventions were not fun places to be. Traditionally these conventions were large, congenial affairs where patients, their families, treatment professionals, and, of course, the fractionators all converged to elect national officers, hear exciting news of medical breakthroughs, eat at lavish banquets and other social events sponsored by the fractionators, and attend seminars on all aspects of hemophilia. The 1992 Atlanta Convention and especially the 1993 convention in Indianapolis, however, are remembered very differently by those who attended. These conventions were scarred with the specter of death and rife with contention.

The November 1992 conference, dubbed "Hot'lanta" by COTT editorial member Tom Fahey, saw the beginning of open protests and major NHF policy shifts in response to outspoken activists. Protestors carried signs outside the convention center and, wearing death masks, angrily confronted fractionators in the commercial exhibit area. Within the conference halls, the NHF made two important concessions to angry activists. The first related to the issue of expert testimony

by NHF-associated doctors. Responding to the anger of people who had unsuccessfully attempted to sue the fractionators and had seen MASAC doctors rise in
support of defendant (i.e., fractionator) claims, the NHF passed a resolution that
physicians associated with NHF should not testify on behalf of fractionators.[56]
Similarly, the NHF also addressed the issue of compensation by government and
the blood industry by setting up its SAC.

These concessions did little to stem the ire of activists, however, and the
1993 Indianapolis conference was, if anything, even more contentious. In 1992 AIDS
was beginning to be recognized by attendees and the NHF as a serious issue; in
1993 it was *the* issue. The NHF had set aside a room filled with quilt panels from
the NAMES Project AIDS Memorial Quilt in memory of men and boys with hemophilia who had died of AIDS. Whole families, parents and children alike, openly
demonstrated outside and within the conference, many sporting black cloaks and
death masks and carrying signs arguing that the NHF itself had betrayed its constituents. At a "town meeting" to discuss the efforts of the SAC, which had been
formed the year before, all hell broke loose. In many ways, SAC had been on shaky
ground from the beginning. COTT and the H/HIV Peer Association objected to its
charity-based approach (asking for financial aid, rather than demanding financial
retribution) and the fact that the lion's share of the proposed contributions would
not go directly to consumers but into a fund that would be administered according
to petitioner's "needs." Industry, on the other hand, objected to the high price tag—
$1.5 billion—and the timing because the IOM investigation was about to begin.[57]
When NHF officers walked into the town meeting with the offers that several individual fractionators had made, the response was loud and angry. H/HIV Peer Association leader Michael Rosenberg denounced the NHF and announced that activists who had given up on SAC and filed their own class action suit were adding the
NHF itself as a defendant in the suit.[58] Attendees cheered the activists of the Peer
Association and openly accused the NHF of all kinds of betrayals—from not providing support when HIV-positive hemophiliacs had been discriminated against to har-
boring doctors who testified against HIV-positive hemophiliacs in their lawsuits
against the fractionators.

The class action suit that Rosenberg spoke of at the October 1993 meeting,
Wadleigh v. Rhone Poulenc, had been filed on September 30, 1993, in federal district court in Chicago. Just as Rosenberg had said, it was filed against the four fractionators as well as the NHF. One of the most important procedures that a class
action lawsuit must undergo is a process called certification. For plaintiffs to be
certified as a class, a judge must decide that four conditions have been met. First,
the class must be so large that individual litigation would be too unwieldy
(numerosity). Second, there must be common issues of law and fact among the
cases (commonality). Third, the claims of the class representatives must be typical
of the claims of the entire class (typicality). Finally, the class representatives must
fairly protect the interests of the class. Not surprisingly (given its position as a defendant in the suit), the NHF opposed certification of the class. Among other arguments, the NHF opposed the commonality issue, arguing that the laws regarding
blood liability are different in all fifty states and that different HIV infections were

caused by different products.[59] Despite these and other arguments, almost a year after the class action was filed Judge John Grady granted the class certification.

Seven months later, however, hemophilia activists were dealt a major blow. Federal Appeals Court Judge Richard Posner took the unusual action of reversing the lower court and decertifying the class. In his decision, Posner highlighted several issues, including concerns that the class action could "hurl an industry into bankruptcy."[60] This fear was compounded by his concern that the class action, though strong on human appeal, was weak in legal merit—an assumption he based on the defendants' 92.3 percent victory record.

The decertification added another layer of turmoil on an already-turbulent situation. At this point, hemophilia activists and their lawyers found themselves at a major impasse. The activists wanted to appeal the Posner decision to the Supreme Court. On the other hand, their lawyers, led by David Shrager, wanted to turn their attention to the individual lawsuits that had been consolidated separate of the class action. To the activists, this strategy was a major sell-out because it would mean that all HIV-positive hemophiliacs who had not filed individual suits because of lack of financial means or other resources, but who had been automatically covered as members of the class, would wind up with nothing. Things got so bad that COTT went to court in an attempt to get rid of the lawyers who were litigating the cases. The attempt was denied, with Judge Grady arguing that it would be like passengers taking control of a plane in mid-flight.[61] Disgusted with the attorneys, COTT leader Corey Dubin went so far as to meet secretly and begin negotiations with one of the four fractionators, Baxter (owner of Miles/Hyland).

Ultimately, the individual negotiations were abandoned and the class action suit was recertified for the express purpose of having it settled out of court. The four companies together agreed to a settlement that amounted to approximately $670 million. The majority of this amount—about $600 million, or $100,000 per claimant (or the claimant's closest family survivor)—went to individual HIV-infected hemophiliacs. Approximately $40 million covered legal fees. An issue that nearly scuttled the deal involved Medicaid and welfare benefits. States that had been paying through Medicaid for the treatment of HIV-infected patients wanted reimbursement, and activists were concerned that patients on welfare might lose their benefits because of the $100,000 payout. The defendant companies kicked in an approximately $30 million ($12 million to the federal government and $18 million to state governments and private insurers) to cover the reimbursement problem, and they created a special-needs fund for welfare recipients that would not endanger their benefits.[62]

Of course, not everyone was happy with the deal. To many if not most activists within the hemophilia community, the deal was an insulting statement that their lives and those of their loved ones could be bought off at $100,000 apiece. It also did not escape the notice of many activists that between factor and their AIDS medicines, many HIV infected hemophiliacs were being forced to buy more than $100,000 worth of pharmaceutical products a year (although most of these drugs were covered by some form of insurance). It also was galling to many that some of the same companies they had settled with had reached a settlement with Japanese hemophiliacs for $420,000 per person. Given these and other factors, many plaintiffs chose not to enter into the settlement at all. These "opt-outs," including most of the leadership of COTT, denounced the deal and chose to take their chances pursuing individual lawsuits. Again, this development nearly brought down the entire settlement. Initially, the four fractionators had agreed to a settlement under the condition that if there were 100 or more opt-outs, the deal was off. Later the companies agreed to modify that position; ultimately, approximately 6,200 took the deal, and several hundred opted out. The opt-outs have continued to pursue their individual cases; in October 2000 a settlement for an undisclosed amount was reached between the four fractionators and most of the remaining opt-outs.[63]

In addition to pursuing the litigation against the private pharmaceutical companies that produce AHF, hemophilia activists have worked to pass legislation that would force the government to pay compensation for its part in their infections. The vehicle for this struggle was the Ricky Ray Hemophilia Relief Act, which was introduced in Congress on February 23, 1995. Representative Porter Goss (R-Fla.) introduced the bill, which was named after a fifteen-year-old constituent with hemophilia who had died of AIDS. Goss's cause gained credibility when the IOM released its report in July 1995.

The bill Goss introduced in February 1995 would have set up a billion dollar fund from which infected hemophiliacs could have claimed a total of $125,000 each, with a sunset date five years after the bill's implementation. Despite the moral boost of the IOM report, the bill went nowhere, and Goss was forced to reintroduce it in the 105th Congress on March 11, 1997, as H.R. 1023, the Ricky Ray Hemophilia Relief Fund of 1998. Goss and the hemophilia community were forced to lower their expectations the second time around—with somewhat better results. The bill asked for only $100,000 per claimant, bringing the total cost of the proposed relief fund down to $750 million. Putting this amount in context, the Judiciary Committee report that accompanied the bill noted that the average *annual* medical cost for an HIV-positive person with hemophilia was $168,480. Significantly, the new bill also explicitly deleted the fault-finding portions of the original bill, noting instead merely that "this community needs humanitarian assistance."[64] The bill did considerably better this time around, passing the full House by voice vote on May 19, 1998.

Of course, one of the truisms of politics is that nothing moves forward without being pushed, and the bill's passage on the House side occurred in no small measure because of the sustained pushing of grassroots members of the hemophilia community. Initially, COTT relied on its own leadership, particularly Dana Kuhn (who lived in Virginia), to lobby Congress. As the burden on the leadership—which itself was struggling with hemophilia and HIV infection—increased, however, COTT invested in full-time lobbyist David Cavanaugh, whose office doubled as an overnight center for community members who flew in from around the country to talk to their own senators and members of Congress. Cavanaugh's efforts were aided by awareness-raising campaigns coordinated by Jan Hamilton, director of the Hemophilia Federation of America, and Kim Bernstein of the Olsten ACCESS Company, a health care advocacy group. These campaigns were designed to emphasize the personal impact of AIDS on the hemophilia community by using visual props such as banners, footsteps (encouraging members of Congress to walk in the shoes of people affected), and hourglasses (large replicas filled with petitions to remind Congress that time was running out). Similarly, several high school students belonging to the Distributive Education Clubs of America (DECA) club of Robinson High School in Fairfax, Virginia, became involved and followed the legislation every year, organizing lobbying days and vigils to keep the issue alive. Perhaps most crucial were lobbying days that were well-attended by hemophilia activists and their survivors who came to Washington, often in their wheelchairs, to share their stories with their representatives.

Most of these efforts were aided by the work Michael Davon did in bringing the hemophilia community into cyberspace. In addition to the e-mail list serve that he set up, he also used his Internet company, the Web-Depot, to host the first hemophilia home page, a bulletin board, and chat rooms. The electronic list was especially important because through this list COTT and the Hemophilia Federation of America were able to post to their membership on a daily basis, if necessary. This capability opened the way for all sorts of coordinated lobbying and awareness actions that helped promote the hemophilia political agenda.

On the Senate side, however, the Ricky Ray bill met with opposition from an unexpected source. After passing the House it was sent, as a health-related bill, to the Senate Committee on Health, Education, Labor and Pensions (HELP). The chair of this committee, Jim Jeffords of Vermont, had a major problem with the bill. His position was that the bill was unfair because it would compensate only hemophiliacs infected with blood products; it would do nothing for the more diffuse group of people who had been infected with HIV through blood transfusions. COTT's position was that both communities would be best served by passing the Ricky Ray bill first and then combining efforts to push through a separate second bill for transfusion-acquired cases in the next Congress. By this juncture a small group, the National Association for Victims of Transfusion-Acquired AIDS (NAVTA), had organized itself to press its own claim. This group, founded by Steven Grissom of Cary, North Carolina, did not have the history or level of shared experience that the HIV/hemophilia community did, but it did appear to have a champion in the office of Jim Jeffords.

For the hemophilia community, Jeffords's challenge came at an inopportune time. Congress works on a two-year calendar: A bill must be passed within the two-year period of a particular Congress (in this case, the 105th) or begin again in the next two-year session. The Ricky Ray bill languished in Jeffords' committee from June 16 to October 7, 1998, when—as a result of intense negotiations between the offices of Jeffords and the bill's chief Senate ally, Mike DeWine (R-Ohio)—it was released from committee to be considered by the full Senate. As a condition of release it was accompanied by a second version written by Jeffords, who wanted to attempt to find sufficient support for his version to substitute it for the original.

An additional timing problem arose at this point, however. When Jeffords released the bill (October 1998) it was hardly high on the list of Senate priorities. This would be true at that time in any two-year legislative cycle. The Senate was eager to conclude its session and recess until Congress reconvened in January. There was an even bigger distraction in fall 1998, however. The Lewinsky scandal was the most important issue on Capitol Hill and was deflecting attention from most other legislative activities. Then, as the rest of Washington's attention was riveted on discovering the ins and outs of the affair between President Clinton and intern Monica Lewinsky, Jeffords tried a new tactic. Using a special power given only to U.S. Senators, he placed a "hold" on the bill, thereby ensuring that it would not be acted on by the full Senate. The hemophilia community threw itself into the struggle with an onslaught of phone calls, faxes, and letters from grassroots members to their Congressional representatives. They also worked with NAVTA's Steven Grissom, who issued a statement to the effect that the transfusion-acquired group would rather delay their claims than see both versions die. In the face of these efforts Jeffords relented, and the bill was passed by unanimous consent literally at the eleventh hour, on the last day of the session (October 21, 1998). On November 12, 1998, in the presence of Ricky Ray's mother, Louise, President Clinton signed it as Public Law 105-369.

This law was not the last word, however, for the hemophilia community or for those with transfusion-acquired AIDS. The hemophilia community was about to learn a bitter lesson about the way congressional funding works—namely, that authorization and appropriation are two separate processes. The Ricky Ray law had created an authorization to pay up to $750 million (or $100,000 per claimant). It was up to the next Congress to actually appropriate the money, however, and according to the way the bill was written, the appropriation had to happen in the succeeding four years or the bill would expire. The community would find, to its chagrin, that it is politically much easier to achieve an authorization than an appropriation. Despite continuing efforts by COTT and its allies, by summer 2000 Congress had appropriated only $75 million—one-tenth of the original amount authorized. HHS, the department charged with actually dispensing the funds, set up a lottery-type system among eligible recipients to determine who would receive a $100,000 check. In fall 2000 the budget process was delayed for six weeks because of elections, Thanksgiving, and the infamous election recounts, leaving Congress three weeks to finish negotiating the fiscal year 2001 budget with outgoing President Clinton. As the result of extensive negotiations (and strong last-minute lobbying from COTT and the grassroots community), Congress in its final Omnibus Funding package appropriated the additional $575 million that was considered the minimum necessary to cover claims.[65]

As for NAVTA and the people for whom it advocates, there has been progress of a very incomplete form. On November 16, 1999, Senator Jeffords had introduced a new bill, which he named the Ricky Ray Fairness Act of 1999. The purpose of this bill was to amend the Ricky Ray Hemophilia Relief Fund Act to include people who acquired HIV through contaminated blood or tissues and were not covered under the original law. The bill was referred to Jeffords's own committee for consideration, but like all such "in-process" legislation it died at the end of the 106th Congress. Jeffords' office had indicated that he had plans to reintroduce the legislation during the 107th Congress,[66] but as of late December 2001 there is no record of this reintroduction in the *Congressional Record,* and it remains to be seen whether Congress will choose to compensate people who were infected with HIV in transfusion cases.

Hemophilia activists pursued calls for investigation that resulted in the IOM study and report. They pursued justice through compensation, which ended in a settlement with the four fractionators for most of the community, as well as passage of the Ricky Ray Act. Like many other AIDS activists, however, they had a third goal— less flashy, perhaps, than the previous ones but enormously important for policymaking. That third goal was *representation*. It was always a central tenant of hemophilia activists that the tragedy of HIV infections within the community could have been avoided if only informed consumers had been given a serious voice in the debates over blood safety to begin with. In this area, activists have effected substantial change.

A first crucial step was taken in May 1994, when hemophilia activists convinced Senators Bob Graham (D-Fla.) and John Glenn (D-Ohio), as well as Representative Goss, to petition the FDA to add a voting role for consumers on the powerful BPAC. The existing committee was opposed to the idea, arguing that the FDA should continue its usual policy of not allowing consumers on any of its advisory committees because they are unable to grasp the difficult technical issues of the subject area.[67] The hemophilia activists prevailed, however, and in 1995 COTT president Corey Dubin became the first grassroots consumer to be named as a voting member of the BPAC, where he began to vigorously promote consumer issues. When his term expired in 2000, he was replaced by COTT board member Terry Rice, thereby ensuring that consumer voting status was not a one-time deal.

The trend of representation that began with the BPAC was replicated when HHS created a new group, the Advisory Committee on Blood Safety and Availability (ACBSA). This new group began its work April 1997 in response to recommendations in the IOM report, and this time consumers had a voice from the start. In addition to Dana Kuhn, representing COTT, Larry Allen—a health activist representing people with sickle cell disease—also was named to the committee.

This last development has been fostered by the creation in 1997 by COTT of a Plasma Users Coalition (PUC), bringing together representatives of several groups whose members use blood products and components and therefore have a stake in the safety of these products. Larry Allen, who sits on the ACBSA, also is a representative of the sickle cell community in the PUC. As these leaders of consumer-based groups work together, they are able to find common ground as consumers who perform a watchdog function relative to producers. A final ambitious but still-unrealized goal of COTT is to require that all FDA advisory committees be required to contain one-third consumer membership. In this way, hemophilia activists hope to help ensure that future catastrophes like the HIV infection of the blood supply in the United States will be averted.

Conclusion

The twin goals of an effective blood policy are to provide a supply of blood and blood products that are adequate and safe. There are strong pressures on the nonprofit blood industry to provide an adequate supply of blood and on the for-profit blood industry to maximize financial gains. The industry, in turn, has pressured the FDA not to be too stringent in its rules regarding the screening, procurement, and processing of blood and blood products. Until the 1980s, this strategy of placing supply over safety appeared to work for everyone concerned, and relationships between the blood industry, its regulators, and consumers were cordial. The disastrous HIV (and hepatitis) contamination of the blood supply has served as a harsh reminder, however, that the needs and agendas of consumers and suppliers often are at odds. In response to their HIV infections, consumers have organized and demanded that the blood industry and its regulators respond to their concerns about safety and justice. The result has been a great deal more conflict between the blood industry, regulators, and consumers. For activists mobilized by the contamination of the blood supply, however, that is a small price to pay in the pursuit of safety and restitution.

In a larger policy context, the struggle over blood supply and safety issues highlights several broader policy features. The actions of the blood industry to avoid additional regulation are the predictable outcome of the desire of all groups in the policy process to evade the infliction of costs. Usually, as in this case, the presumption is with well-organized commercial interests such as the blood industry unless and until a disaster occurs, illustrating to everyone the need for more regulation. This case also illustrates the power of organization, even when individuals have far fewer resources at their disposal than the groups against which they are organizing. When the small but well-bonded hemophilia community organized against the much more heavily resourced blood industry, that community was able to achieve several policy aims, including compensatory legislation. By contrast, the lack of strong organization on the part of the larger collection of transfusion-related HIV-positive individuals has strongly hindered similar efforts for that community.

CHAPTER 4

Dueling Models of AIDS Prevention: Harm Reduction and Abstinence

On October 14, 1987, conservative Republican Jesse Helms opened a national debate over how best to prevent the spread of HIV with a passionate appeal to his colleagues on the Senate floor. Indignant with anger, he waved a comic book that had been written and distributed by GMHC in New York City. The book depicted a casual but "safer" (that is, condom-using) sexual encounter between two men. Incensed by the book, Helms said he had confronted GMHC, and the organization had responded that "federal dollars [were] not being used to produce this material." The money was used, however, for a series of workshops and educational session that were designed to provide "AIDS risk reduction education."[1] Helms went on to describe some of the workshops envisioned in the two-year grant, including "Gay Identity Roles and Sexuality," Social Skills Development," "Guidelines for Safer Sex," and "Dating and Intimacy." His description was punctuated by frequent personal appraisals of the supposed futility and revolting nature of the project, and he concluded that only educational materials promoting abstinence—from homosexual activity, intravenous drug use, or any sexual activity outside of monogamous heterosexual marriage—were appropriate. To further the goal of providing such appropriate materials, he offered a provision, Amendment 956, that would have prohibited the CDC from using any government-authorized funds to "provide AIDS education, information, or prevention materials and activities that promote, encourage or condone sexual activity outside a sexually monogamous marriage (including homosexual activities) or the use of intravenous drugs."[2]

Senator Helms is well known for his opposition toward behaviors and groups that he considers to be a threat to his concept of "family values," so his position on this particular day was not surprising. More notable is the fact that he drew almost no verbal opposition from his more liberal colleagues in the Senate. At the time, only two voices rose to challenge him, and their messages were not united. The stronger words came from fellow Republican Lowell Weicker. After carefully distancing himself and the federal government from the offending comic book, he argued that education and research were, at the time, the only weapons available for fighting the emerging epidemic. He claimed, therefore, that "any sort of an education process that excludes a part of the population, in particular a high-risk population, is not the education effort that the crisis deserves."[3]

The other source of opposition was less emphatic. Senator Lawton Chiles, a Democrat from Florida, first dismissed Weicker's concerns about at-risk gay men with the comment, "I guess you can say that as long as this disease is confined among homosexuals, no real danger." Chiles's concern was for the heterosexuals who might become infected through intravenous drug use and then pass on the virus through heterosexual intercourse. This prospect was worrisome because "that is getting into my neighborhood. That is getting into where it can be involved with people that I know and love and care about, and that is where it is getting to children."[4] Senator Chiles's argument apparently struck a chord because Helms's amendment ultimately was modified to only prohibit funding efforts that would seem to be promoting homosexuality.

More than five years later, unbeknownst to Senator Helms, others would find themselves debating the issue that he had sacrificed to get part of his amendment passed. The scene had shifted from the floor of the Senate to a packed conference room in Boston. An argument was raging among community activists sitting on a panel titled "The Impact of Syringe Exchange on Communities of Color," and the question was not whether to help gay men reduce their health risks while maintaining their sex lives. In this forum the issue was whether and how to allow people to reduce their risks while managing their drug habits. As the panel went back and forth over the pros and cons of providing clean needles to active addicts, the audience and panelists became increasingly agitated. Finally one of the panelists, a man named Gregory Davis, could stand it no longer. "No needle exchange!" he shouted. "Not now, not ever in this city!" With that parting shot he stormed out of the room.

These two confrontations involved different spokespeople, different communities, different forums, even different subjects, but the underlying core issue was the same. What was and remains at stake in the field of AIDS prevention is a clash between two competing strategies. Although Senator Helms and Mr. Davis likely have next to nothing else in common, they are both adherents to a strategy of *abstinence*. As the term implies, abstinence proponents seek to have at-risk individuals discontinue entirely the sexual or drug-using practices that create possible risks for the spread of HIV. In contrast, the competing strategy of *harm or risk reduction* assumes that people may continue the core sexual or drug using behaviors that put them at risk. The focus for adherents of the harm reduction model is on finding ways to encourage people to conduct these behaviors in a way that minimizes the risks that come with them. The policy struggles around preventing the spread of HIV infection often vary according to specific times, places, and risk groups, but they usually include some element of contention over which core strategy (abstinence or harm reduction) is more desirable.

As the epidemic has progressed, one important and continuous finding has been that HIV is not transmitted casually. Mosquitoes, hugging, sneezing, toilet seats—none of these has ever been implicated in a case of HIV transmission. The three main routes of HIV transmission (all involving the exchange of body fluids) are sexual contact, needles and syringes, and mother-to-child.[5] Given that there are so few means of transmission, that the means of transmission are known, and that we do not have an effective vaccine or a medical cure, the goal of prevention becomes extraordinarily important. Prevention of HIV transmission is based on the concept of behavior modification—that is, on convincing people not to engage in behaviors that enable HIV to be transmitted. This observation, however, brings us back to the abstinence/harm reduction conflict. Is it better to convince people not to engage in certain behaviors at all (abstinence) or to teach them ways of engaging in behaviors in such a way as to minimize the risk of HIV transmission while the behavior is occurring?

The disagreement over these two strategies stems in part from a more fundamental disagreement about certain core behaviors, particularly drug use and sexual activity outside of heterosexual marriage. Most proponents of abstinence believe that these behaviors are wrong and themselves are the problem to be solved. According to this train of thought, HIV transmission is simply an indicator of a deeper evil. Harm reduction adherents do not regard drug use or various types of sexual encounters as bad in themselves. The harm occurs, they argue, because of the way in which the behavior is conducted. Thus, the problems of pregnancy, AIDS, and other sexually transmitted diseases all occur when sex is performed "unsafely." Similarly, drug use is problematic not for its mood-altering effects but because of the health problems (e.g., AIDS and hepatitis) and social problems (e.g., theft and prostitution) that occur when drug use becomes uncontrollable.

Although both strategies are offered as solutions to the problem of HIV transmission, they usually are regarded (especially by abstinence promoters) as mutually exclusive. The concept of abstinence is based on several absolute premises. The harm reduction model views behaviors along a continuum and promotes any modification of behavior that decreases the risk of transmission as progress. In contrast, abstinence models rely on complete compliance for their success. Thus, harm reduction proponents regard abstinence as just one alternative (although it is often discounted as a judgmental approach) in the large range of options for decreasing risk behaviors. For supporters of abstinence, harm reduction approaches fundamentally undermine the intent and effectiveness of their programs.

Politically, each of these approaches has been backed by an initial community or set of policymakers. These initial groups gathered larger coalitions to help in their struggles. Harm reduction was initiated by activists and AIDS organizations in the gay community as an attempt to educate and warn its at-risk population without touching off a wave of anger and denial. As these initial actors and organizations took their messages and strategies outside the gay community, they found allies among many public health officials (who often already had embraced harm reduction's assumptions in their professional work), civil libertarians, and advocates and organizations for reproductive rights such as Planned Parenthood.

Abstinence models, on the other hand, initially received public support from conservative politicians and Christian fundamentalist and Catholic religious leaders. As the issue of AIDS reanimated old causes, this core coalition attracted additional support from parents who were concerned about their own loss of control over the information their children were receiving. Leadership also was provided by many churches and abstinence-based drug treatment programs within minority—particularly African-American—communities.

The struggle over these seemingly incompatible approaches has had far-reaching (at times even crippling) consequences for AIDS prevention workers. One of the most visible examples of an AIDS educator who learned the hard way about the lack of a middle ground in this debate was C. Everett Koop, U.S. Surgeon General from 1981 to 1989. Koop entered the AIDS arena with deep personal convictions that closely mirrored those of the abstinence advocates. He was strongly opposed to drug use and extramarital sex of any kind, and he considered the anal intercourse practiced by many gay men and some heterosexuals "a violation of laws both spiritual and temporal."[6] Yet his early determination that his role as Surgeon General was to save lives led him to advocacy, however qualified, of two policies that were strongly opposed by his conservative former allies within and outside the White House. Koop always described these policies—broad-based sex education within the schools and condom distribution—as second-best strategies that had been necessitated by the breakdown of traditional family values in American society.

Yet all of these qualifications and disclaimers were lost on advocates of harm reduction and abstinence alike. Both groups viewed Koop as squarely within the harm reduction camp and criticized or hailed him accordingly. This consistent oversimplification was a source of constant frustration to Koop, who described the dynamic as follows:

> I never mentioned the use of condoms as a preventative measure against AIDS without *first* stressing the much better and safer alternatives of *abstinence* and *monogamy*. I also said that condoms were all we had to offer but that they were not 100 percent reliable, although they were often more reliable than the people who used them. Often I would spend several minutes of a speech extolling abstinence and monogamy (for social and moral reasons as well as reasons of health), and then at the end I would say that those foolish enough not to practice abstinence or mutually faithful monogamy should, for their protection and their partner's protection, use a latex condom. Usually the press would repeat only the last phrase. That annoyed me.[7]

Faced with a no-win situation, Koop eventually threw caution to the wind and allied himself with his former foes (who had bitterly and vocally opposed his nomination as surgeon general). His massive mailing of a six-page AIDS prevention pamphlet titled "Understanding AIDS: A Message from the Surgeon General" to 107 million Americans in 1988 cemented his position as a "traitor" to the abstinence camp (to which he still personally belonged). Among the specific pieces of advice in this pamphlet was the statement that "condoms are the best preventative measure against AIDS besides not having sex and practicing safe behavior." A section on drug use noted that "many drug users are addicted and need to enter a treatment program as quickly as possible. In the meantime, these people must avoid AIDS by not sharing any of the equipment used to prepare and inject illegal drugs."[8]

Although these admonitions were hardly sex or drug-positive messages, and other parts of the pamphlet (such as the lists of "risky" and "safe" behaviors) clearly cast abstinence in a very positive light, the perceived value neutrality of at least portions of the pamphlet were enough to permanently consign Koop to the ranks of the harm reductionists for the remainder of his term as Surgeon General.

These competing prevention strategies often are represented as the sides in a debate between pragmatism (harm reduction) and idealism (abstinence). This representation regards harm reduction as a "do what you must to save lives" strategy, as opposed to the abstinence model's underlying goal of preservation of a traditional "family values" culture. This view, however, obscures the fact that harm reduction, in the initial form of safer sex messages, was adopted by the gay community not only to save lives but also to preserve a distinctive, sex-positive culture.

As prevention models have evolved to address the specific needs of a spectrum of at-risk groups, the array of strategies and controversies has grown immensely. Comprehensive coverage of these ideas and debates would require a book in itself. Therefore, as in other chapters in this volume, I use a more limited approach. Policymakers have envisioned ways of blocking HIV transmission in each of the three major transmission routes—sexual contact, needles and syringes, and mother-to-child—and in this chapter I examine one prevention strategy for each case.

Although safer sex messages have their roots in the gay community, one of their most controversial "transplantings" has occurred in the attempt to fashion effective AIDS education and condom distribution programs in public schools. Thus, the first of my three case studies examines this process of creating the safer sex strategy and then implementing it in public schools. Because this process has been very localized, with results varying widely according to local values, I do not attempt to discuss how these policy struggles have played out in all school districts across the country. Instead, I focus on the largest and one of the most controversial and widely reported cases: the New York City school district.

As with AIDS education and condom distribution, the most widely discussed prevention strategy for drug users—needle exchange—has been extremely controversial. It also has been fought over primarily at the local level, and results again have varied widely, depending on the values of the people of particular states and municipalities. Therefore I focus on the site of the nation's largest drug-using population, which also happens to be one of the most controversial and well-reported cases: New York City.

I return to New York (the entire state this time) for the third case study. The third major route of transmission of HIV is from mother to child, which may occur in utero, during birth, or from breast feeding. In this case I depart somewhat from the harm reduction-abstinence fight to a conflict that is framed around privacy rights and fetal protections. Like the other cases I examine, this one is enormously controversial, and it involves moral and practical dimensions.

Can Safer Sex Be a Universal Solution?

Although it would be hard to find a person who is *opposed* to preventing the transmission of HIV, the consensus surrounding the desirability of prevention immediately breaks down when the project of converting ideas to action begins. The first educational messages were generated from within the gay community—most significantly, from newly created AIDS service organizations. In trying to determine the content of these messages, the earliest such organization, GMHC, faced the difficult challenge of educating an unreceptive audience with information that was highly incomplete, at best. The initial warnings of a new disease spreading among gay men in San Francisco, Los Angeles, and New York City were met with denial and anger within the gay community, even though the messages were delivered by members of that same community.

One of the earliest such warnings came from playwright Larry Kramer, who was a founding member of GMHC and ACT UP/New York. He began to write about an epidemic in fall 1981, before it even had a name. Kramer used the pages of the weekly *New York Native* to put forward his unpopular and emotional message—and was branded alarmist and homophobic for his trouble.[9]

The linkage between having numerous sexual partners and the disease came from outside the gay community, specifically epidemiologists; yet the link also was discussed within the community by gay physicians with practices serving many of the earliest AIDS patients. The most well-known of these physicians was Joe Sonnabend, whose work also was crucial to the founding and early success of the American Foundation for AIDS Research (AmFAR) and the Community Research Initiative. Sonnabend argued (before the discovery of HIV) that it was "promiscuity itself, together with the attendant multiple and repeated bouts of sexually transmitted diseases that produced such catastrophic clinical results."[10] Several of Sonnabend's patients, particularly Michael Callen, adopted Sonnabend's ideas and argued them even more forcefully in the pages of the gay press.[11]

As the controversy went back and forth, GMHC decided as a group (over the strenuous objection of board member Larry Kramer) that it should provide the most up-to date-information to gay men and allow them to decide what to do with it. To implement this decision, GMHC used its publications to offer varying views on risk reduction. These views ran the gamut from those of a sociologist who argued that there was, in fact, no epidemic going on to suggestions (still arguably mild in the face of a fatal disease) that gay men might consider having fewer sexual partners and choosing partners who appeared to be in good health.[12]

Throughout this period (1981 through early 1983), the CDC and various researchers continued to compile data suggesting that HIV moved through the exchange of bodily fluids—primarily blood, semen, and vaginal secretions.[13] Although the mainstream media rarely covered AIDS issues until the death of Rock Hudson in 1985, the gay community was keeping up with epidemiological and medical developments by monitoring the scientific literature on the emerging epidemic.

As more knowledge on how HIV is spread became available, there was an important shift in the missions of most AIDS service organizations. As the consensus in the medical community grew around the transmissibility of HIV through unprotected sex, the "present-all-sides-but-draw-no-conclusions" strategy seemed to be increasingly unethical. This was particularly true because the gay community (like every subsequent community that was forced to face the epidemic) was in an initial period of denial. The question shifted from *whether* to warn people about the danger of "unsafe" sex to *how* to provide such a warning in a way that was accessible and gay-positive.

The broad answer was the concept of "safer sex" (initially referred to as "safe sex"). The safer sex message promoted the idea that the key to maintaining an HIV-negative status lay in decreasing one's risk of transferring bodily fluids.

Rather than promoting abstinence from any particular type of sexual contact, the message promoted the use of condoms (or other barrier methods such as dental dams) during sex.

Getting the word out required that this message be taken to places where at-risk gay men were sexually and socially active and that the message itself be delivered in understandable and community-friendly ways. Given these needs, the content of pamphlets and other educational materials and messages designed to educate sexually active gay men was hardly surprising. The materials were written in very explicit (at least by the larger community's standards) terms and tended to depict sexual encounters (provided that they were conducted in a "safer" manner) in a very positive light.

Initially these educational messages sparked little controversy because the funding for their development and their target audience were contained almost completely within the gay community. As the spread of AIDS continued at an increasingly rapid pace, however (and as everyone began to realize that gay men were not the only people turning up HIV-positive), the community-based organizations began to turn to the state and the larger society for support. With this support came increasing scrutiny, which in turn led to outrage on the part of conservative politicians.

"Community norms" of sexually active members of the gay community were not easily reconciled with the moral beliefs of conservative local and national officials. Jesse Helms's tirade on the floor of the Senate was only one notable incident in a wave of public backlash over the perception that public funding was being used to condone sexual acts that were technically criminal in half the states. A similar controversy erupted when a member of the Los Angeles County Board of Supervisors was shown a copy of the brochure "Mother's Handy Sex Guide," which had been distributed in 1985 by AIDS Project Los Angeles with at least some state funding.[14] The brochure contained an explicit cover photograph (a man clad only in an athletic supporter), very direct language, and stories of gay male sexual fantasies describing "safer" sexual encounters. The offended board member characterized the brochure as pornography rather than educational material. The state of California's response to the controversy was the establishment of a Materials Review Committee that set up guidelines to control the explicit content of educational materials distributed by publicly funded groups. Content developers were advised to substitute "clinical or descriptive terms" rather than their "slang or street language equivalents" and to keep visual content from being "explicitly suggestive."[15]

Ultimately, the CDC itself tackled the same problem, and in 1986 it issued its compromise solution: Local panels would be convened to review any CDC-funded educational materials developed by local AIDS organizations. State and local health officials would approve the membership of the panels, and certain guiding principles would be followed:

> The terms used in all educational materials were to be understandable by those to whom it was directed but not offensive when judged by a "reasonable person." Pictorial material was to avoid the display of the "anogenital area of the body" or overt depiction of the performance of "safer sex" or "unsafe" sex practices.[16]

The level of controversy over educational materials that were developed and directed within the gay community was nothing, however, compared to the firestorm in the larger society over educational outreach efforts targeted at adolescents a few years later. Although various elected officials and religious and civic leaders occasionally railed against educational efforts that—with or without public funding—promoted a "perverted" way of life, prevention education within the gay community was regarded largely as an issue for that community. For AIDS activists, this attitude was a blessing and a curse. One the positive side, AIDS educators continued (though they sometimes were limited to private sources of funding) to advocate prevention methods tailored to the specific needs and desires of various sectors of the at-risk gay community. On the other hand, such efforts denied the medical reality that gay white men, for whom the majority of education was being developed, were not the only ones at risk. This emphasis also dampened the larger community's willingness to support AIDS service organizations because the perception was that this educational effort was an obligation primarily for the gay community. It was not surprising, therefore, when AIDS organizations that were rooted in the gay community decided to branch into prevention efforts beyond the gay community. The decision was based partly on the epidemiological reality that others were at risk and partly on the political reality that AIDS activism would receive a boost if others were made to perceive that risk.

One of the logical targets for these new prevention efforts was teenagers. Teens tend to have multiple sexual partners and, often, unprotected intercourse. These risk behaviors result in approximately three million cases of sexually transmitted diseases and one million pregnancies among teens annually.[17] Research also has shown that only 11 percent of teenagers get most of their information regarding sexually transmitted diseases from parents or other family members.[18]

If teens seemed a logical group to target, the tools for prevention to be employed were not so self-evident. The debate has revolved primarily around three questions. First, are schools the appropriate forum for conducting HIV/AIDS education? Should the educational curriculum focus on an abstinence message or a harm reduction message? Finally, should condom distribution by the schools be included in prevention efforts?

According to a summary issued by the Kaiser Family Foundation in September 2000, some form of sex education is being taught in 95 percent of public schools in the United States.[19] This number, however, masks the extraordinary complexity of forms such education may take. Some states mandate general sex education; others specify HIV or sexually transmitted disease (STD) education. In fact, thirty-four states mandate HIV/STD education, but only eighteen require general sex education!

The specific mandates also vary widely. Some states require abstinence-only education that teaches abstinence until marriage as the only alternative. Others offer comprehensive or "abstinence-plus" curricula that provide information about abstinence and risk reduction while advocating abstinence as the preferred option. To complicate matters further, among states that do not require sex education, many have stipulations that *if* sex education is taught it must have certain components—such as abstinence-until-marriage instructions.[20] States with abstinence-only policies tend to be silent on questions of prevention for same-gender sexual encounters, although at least one state (North Carolina) specifically addresses these issues as well. In 1996 the North Carolina state board of education, in accordance with a 1995 law, ordered the schools not only to teach that abstinence is the only form of safe sex but that homosexual acts, in addition to transmitting HIV, are illegal.[21]

Matching the diversity of opinion among the states is a similar lack of consensus at the local level. Even states with specific sex and HIV/AIDS education policies often leave the implementation, oversight, and content decisions to local school districts.[22] The decision-making process in many localities has become profoundly political. School board elections have hinged on the issue, and parents have turned out in droves to hotly debate the merits of different prevention and education plans. Coalitions have sprung up in the struggles over local policies, with church and conservative morality groups favoring abstinence-only education, and AIDS service organizations, family planning groups, student organizations, and gay and civil liberties advocates favoring harm reduction and condom distribution programs.

Although the federal government has never explicitly *mandated* national education policies in this area, it has had considerable impact on the issue. Three initiatives have been particularly important. The first, which predated fear of HIV/ AIDS among heterosexual adolescents, was the 1981 Adolescent Family Life Act (AFLA). Funding under this Act, which generally has been in the $6–18 million range annually, was more than doubled to $40 million in fiscal year 2000. The most important stated goal of the legislation was to prevent teen pregnancy by emphasizing self-discipline and chastity. The Act has had a controversial history. Initially AFLA often provided grants to conservative and religious groups that developed abstinence-based curricula. To the American Civil Liberties Union (ACLU), that strategy represented a violation of the separation between church and state; in 1985 a federal court agreed with the ACLU that the Act was unconstitutional. The U.S. Supreme Court reversed the ruling, however, although it remanded the case for further fact-finding. Finally, in 1993, a five-year settlement was reached that kept AFLA-funded programs from making religious references or being conducted in religious settings (including parochial schools). At the expiration of the five-year date, the office that oversees AFLA said that it would continue to use the settlement guidelines in administering the law.[23]

The second initiative, which came from a very different source, was begun by the CDC in 1988. At that time, the CDC released a set of guidelines for AIDS prevention in school health education. The fourteen-page guidelines strongly emphasize an abstinence approach but also admit that "some young people many remain unwilling to adopt behavior that would virtually eliminate their risk of becoming infected." To those people the guidelines recommended (among other things) "using a latex condom with spermicide if they engage in sexual intercourse."[24] Although hardly a ringing endorsement of safer sex, it was more positive toward the concept than the Principles for AIDS Education proposed by the Domestic Policy Council and endorsed by President Reagan in 1987. These principles were appended to the CDC guidelines; they concluded with the guideline that "Any health infor-mation provided by the Federal Government that might be used in schools should teach that children should not engage in sex and should be used with the consent and involvement of parents."[25]

In addition to issuing guidelines, the CDC also began to give out grant money in 1988 to support HIV/STD education in the schools. As the epidemic pro-gressed, the materials in the CDC-supported curriculum became more explicit. By the year 2000, analysts were reporting that opposition to the ongoing grant program had arisen on the basis of objections to the language and materials in the proposed education curriculum.[26]

As for the third major government initiative affecting HIV/STD education, it was tied to welfare reform. In 1996, when Congress passed the Temporary Assis-tance to Needy Families (TANF) Act, it also made available $250 million begin-ning in fiscal year 1998. The money had to be used to promote abstinence-unless-married programs that could be taught as community-based or in-school programs. The provisions of the law mandated very specific teachings about the concept of abstinence. Among the teaching messages required is the idea that any sexual activity that is not conducted within marriage is likely to be physically and psycho-logically harmful.[27]

The federal government's actions in this area illustrate several important policy points. Although the government never required state or local governments to create any particular sort of HIV/STD program, the ability to provide incentives through funding (as well as ready-made curricula and materials that cut down on the work of others) has meant that the federal government has had a significant ability to push education policy in certain directions. This ability has been impeded somewhat, however, by another policy truism: that the federal government does not speak with one voice and that the direction of its voices changes even within a given presidential administration. As the AIDS epidemic has moved through the Reagan, Bush, and Clinton years and into the George W. Bush era, it has been addressed differently by different administrations. Sometimes, as in the Reagan years, differ-ent bureaucracies have responded in different ways.

Ultimately, however, decisions about HIV prevention efforts in the schools are made at the local level. Therefore, to illustrate how the policy struggle plays out in a local arena, I examine one such local battle. As with so many other AIDS-related issues, the policies and processes set in motion in New York City have been instructive for the rest of the country. With regard to the issue of AIDS and adoles-cents, New York City has several dubious distinctions. In addition to having the largest number of diagnosed AIDS cases of any city in the country, it also has 20 percent of the country's thirteen- to twenty-one-year-old cases, among only 3 per-cent of the country's youth population.[28] Moreover, the system charged with the implementation of an HIV prevention program is enormous and complex:

> Authority to manage New York City's public schools, a mammoth
> organization encompassing nearly a million students and a hun-
> dred thousand teachers and staff, is uneasily divided between the

central Board of Education, led by its chancellor, and thirty-two community school districts, each with its own board and its own superintendent. In theory, the central board is legally responsible for matters of "city-wide impact," while the community boards are supposed to attend to local concerns. But the dividing line is far from sharp, and controversies, including court cases, are the norm.[29]

New York City schools were not the first to tackle the issue of AIDS prevention education. Nor were they the first to adopt condoms as part of their AIDS prevention education strategy. That distinction belongs to the Adams County school district in Commerce City, Colorado, which had been distributing condoms district-wide since 1988. What makes New York City stand out—besides the enormity of its system—is the comprehensiveness of the program it implemented in the early 1990s and the level of community involvement that went into its formulation.

New York City went through an arduous process to reach its ambitious educational initiatives, which included a redesigned K–12 curriculum and a condom distribution program run by specially trained HIV/AIDS education teams consisting of volunteer parents, students, and faculty.[30] The school system had dealt with the issue of condom distribution in the past and had briefly allowed the distribution of condoms from school clinics in 1986. That practice ended, however, when several members of the Board of Education—backed by a coalition of ministers, rabbis, and Catholic leaders—opposed the plan.[31]

Between 1986, when the condoms were taken out of the schools, and 1990, when their reintroduction was proposed, AIDS activists attempted to publicize the need for concentrated AIDS prevention efforts among adolescents. ACT UP/New York included the New York City schools in a set of protest activities scheduled for the nationally coordinated Nine Days of Protest that occurred from April 29 to May 7, 1988. On May 4, 1988 (the day directed at women's issues), ACT UP members visited nine different high schools with sexually explicit prevention materials and condoms, dental dams, and lubricants. They talked to students about safer sex, demonstrated how to use the condoms and dental dams, and gave away all the materials they had brought. Activists noted that "apart from the direct intervention, the action also implicitly functioned as a protest of the board of education's refusal to give young people explicit safe information."[32]

ACT UP's own appraisal of the effect of the group's actions was mixed. Members found the teens to be almost uniformly receptive to the information and condom distribution; school officials' reactions varied, however, from those who "proposed formal presentations in the future" to the school principal who "stood at the school's entrance with a garbage can to collect the condoms."[33]

ACT UP may have raised awareness around the issue, but the wheels of change finally began to turn in earnest almost two years later when a subcommittee of the Board of Education's AIDS/HIV Advisory Council requested a meeting with chancellor Joseph A. Fernandez to discuss what subcommittee members perceived as a lack of commitment to prevention efforts.[34] At the subsequent meeting they argued that the need for prevention efforts was urgent and made the case for establishment of a new high-quality curriculum and condom distribution in the schools. A second meeting with the full Advisory Council and the chancellor was held on August 30, 1990. The August meeting also was well attended by groups that perceived themselves as having a stake in the outcome, including AIDS activists and representatives of the Catholic Church. The chancellor announced his intention to adopt all of the Advisory Council's recommendations except condom distribution, which would require further examination. After reviewing information provided in part by the New York City Department of Health, the Chancellor announced his position to support this measure as well.[35]

The next step was the development of a comprehensive HIV/AIDS education plan for all grades, which was accomplished with the aid of an advocacy coalition that included activists, educators, and health professionals. The resulting draft plan was discussed with "labor unions, the Federation of Parent Associations, district and high school superintendents and principals, members of locally elected community school boards, clerical leaders, and advocacy organizations."[36]

Although the issues were still hotly debated, the momentum clearly had shifted. The substance of the debate no longer focused on whether the schools were the appropriate forum for education and condom distribution but on how these activities should be conducted. The membership of the Board of Education had changed; five of the board members in 1990 were different from those of 1986, and four of these new members supported the new measures. In addition, the 1990 board president, Dr. Gwendolynn C. Baker, had switched from her 1986 position opposing condom distribution, saying, "The issue for us is not should we distribute condoms, but how."[37] Similarly, the direction of leadership from the city government had changed, and new mayor David Dinkins had made promises to promote school-based condom distribution to win the endorsement of some women's groups that had faulted mayor Ed Koch on this point.[38]

The HIV/AIDS education program, including condom availability, underwent intense public scrutiny before its final adoption. Written comment was expressly invited from more than 1,000 individuals and groups, and public hearings and meetings were scheduled (one twelve hours long) to air opposing views.

> Citizens spoke about adolescent sexuality and family morals, about religious conviction and the risk of disease, about the breakdown of society and the crime of ignorance. Some speakers asserted that children were dying and others called people who are infected deviants. There were protests and prayer vigils. The newspapers and television news reported the sometimes hysterical and chaotic atmosphere that pervaded the public sessions of the Board.[39]

Although there was outspoken opposition by many parents and the Coalition of Concerned Clergy (which included Catholic, Jewish, Greek Orthodox, and Pentecostal leaders), the results of a citywide survey conducted by the Roper Organization for GMHC indicated that 68 percent of parents favored condom availability in the schools. The school board voted 4 to 3 to adopt the expanded HIV/AIDS program, including its condom availability elements. The decision was strengthened by a 1992 decision by the New York State Supreme Court, which ruled against a school board member and four parents. They had filed a lawsuit against the chancellor and Board of Education claiming that the program violated parental rights of practice of religion and consent for provision of medical services.[40]

Implementation of the new curriculum and condom program carried significant political cost. Although Chancellor Fernandez presided over the program's adoption, it has been widely credited as a cause of his own downfall. In his struggle to install the new plan, the chancellor had angered much of the board, and the situation was worsened by a similar struggle over the so-called rainbow curriculum. This curriculum, which was designed to teach tolerance of racial, religious, and (most controversial) sexual diversity, was championed by Fernandez but again bitterly opposed by elements of the board, as well as some school districts within the system. Finally, in a six-hour session in 1993, the board voted 4 to 3 not to renew the chancellor's contract.[41]

The ouster of Fernandez was followed by a shift away from the sweeping changes he had implemented. His successor, Ramon C. Cortines, revised the school curriculum to emphasize abstinence and allowed parents to "opt-out" their children from prevention discussions.[42] In late 1993 the board replaced many of the members of its AIDS Advisory Council with more conservative members. Among those who were ousted was condom availability advocate and Council cochair Edward McCabe, who angrily editorialized in the *New York Times:*

> The board continually impeded and ignored the curriculum recommendations of its AIDS Advisory Council, and finally replaced many members who had expertise on AIDS or adolescence. As a result, many local districts rely on outdated guidelines from the state, or worse, on the ad hoc policies of community boards. A comprehensive, up-to-date curriculum is available for the elementary grades, but 16 of the 32 districts are not using it because they do not approve of parts of it.[43]

Cortines's tenure as Chancellor was short-lived, however, and in June 1995, after several public exchanges with Mayor Rudolph Giuliani, he quit. His replacement, Rudy Crew—together with the newly reconstituted HIV/AIDS Advisory Council—continued the reversal in policy direction that had begun with the ouster of Fernandez. A new curriculum, backed by Chancellor Crew and Giuliani, eliminated most discussion about gays and lesbians and ended all classroom condom demonstrations. In place of the more comprehensive condom education program, the schools instituted a new policy that would allow private instruction and condom distribution to students who specifically requested them. Such students would go to semi-private resource rooms staffed by trained faculty volunteers during hours determined by the individual school.[44]

Predictably, the changes in policy displeased many people, and in March 1997 students and their allies from various advocacy groups let their discontent be known. In the second week of March, they staged demonstrations in front of more than thirty high schools, arguing that the by-request-only system didn't work for many teens who were too embarrassed to ask for information on condom use. They also accused many of the high schools of not offering the six AIDS prevention classes per year mandated by the Board of Education's health curriculum.[45]

Although the protest did not have the effect of reversing the move of condoms to the resource rooms, proponents of condom availability and risk reduction education received a shot in the arm the following fall with the release of a major new study. The study attempted to examine the long-held suspicion that wide availability of condoms would increase the sexual activity of teens. In the study, students from public high schools in Chicago and New York City during the 1994–95 academic year were compared. Chicago schools offered HIV/AIDS education but no condoms, whereas the New York City schools offered both. Rates of condom use and sexual activity were measured; the researchers found that easy access to condoms did not increase sexual activity, though it did increase condom use.[46]

Like most studies of this nature, the Chicago–New York comparison did not settle the policy controversy because the study was addressing empirical and pragmatic questions, not underlying values. The New York City debate over the role of HIV/AIDS education and condom distribution in the schools continues because it mirrors the societal values debate going on underneath it. The lives of students in the public schools are arguably at stake, but so are deeply held moral and religious convictions of parents and community members. Therefore, the policy battle will not be fought exclusively over the pragmatic question of how to help sexually active teens avoid HIV transmission. Various groups and individuals will go to the mat over moral and religious questions about whether students should be sexually active at all and how our policy choices will affect such behavior.

Saviors of the Sick or Enabling Self-Destruction?

When the gay community attempted to promote sex-positive risk reduction messages from within, outsiders objected. When this same educational approach was tailored to fit an adolescent population, proponents of abstinence launched organizational efforts to counter it. Therefore, controversy was predictable as well when this same risk reduction message was again retooled and introduced as the way to stop, or at least slow, the rampant transmission of HIV among injection drug users and their sexual partners. Fundamentally, risk reduction in the context of drug use means needle exchange, although bleach distribution, expanded access to drug treatment (including methadone maintenance, itself a risk reduction program), and safer sex promotion also figure into the strategy.

At the federal level, the clear message with respect to the problem of HIV transmission through drug use, as well as drug use itself, is that abstinence is the best and only answer. The rhetorical line has been consistent with the "Just Say No" campaign against drug use initiated during the Reagan administration. The federal agency most obviously linked to the issue, the National Institute on Drug Abuse, made its position clear as early as 1985: "NIDA does not feel comfortable sending information which tells drug abusers not to use dirty needles or share needles. NIDA's position is based on [the clear] message, 'Do not use drugs.'"[47] As if to provide an additional exclamation point to its position, NIDA also sent out a formal prohibition to researchers receiving grant funds from the institute in the late 1980s, specifically blocking them from even studying needle-exchange programs.[48]

Since 1988, every Congress and every president has maintained the original ban on federal funding for the actual conduct of needle-exchange programs. In that time, activists have pressured politicians to lift the ban. President Clinton initially endorsed lifting the ban during his 1992 presidential campaign, and an increasing number of organizations and advocacy groups have called for the policy change as well.

> Since 1990, seven national reports have reviewed the scientific evidence and recommended that the federal ban for NEP [Needle Exchange Program] funding be lifted. Needle-exchange programs are supported by the President's Advisory Council on HIV/AIDS, the American Medical Association, the National Academy of Sciences, the Centers for Disease Control and Prevention, and the American Public Health Association, as well as other prestigious medical and public health organizations. In addition, the American Bar Association and the U.S. Conference of Mayors have urged the federal government to allow federal HIV prevention funds to implement NEPs.[49]

On September 17, 1997, another campaign to lift the ban culminated in a demonstration in Washington, D.C., led by ACT UP/Philadelphia and the National Coalition to Save Lives Now. Bearing signs that read, "Moral Backbone for Clinton" and "Moral Backbone for Shalala," the protesters attempted to deliver a twelve-foot replica of a human spine to their targets.[50] According to a *Washington Post* article that was part of a retrospective series on the Clinton presidency, protesters came incredibly close to achieving their aims in the 1997 campaign. Clinton had been ready to unveil a plan to reverse the ban, but then it was "canceled an hour before it was to be announced; consultants said polling showed it could backfire badly with the public."[51]

Yet despite the official embrace of an abstinence posture by many levels of the federal government (with significant exceptions, including the surgeon general and the CDC), harm reductionists at the grassroots level have been remarkably active in promoting and implementing their programs. These programs most often take the form of needle exchanges whereby workers (sometimes volunteers, sometimes professionals, often ex-users) meet with clients to exchange used injection drug syringes for clean ones; they usually offer some mix of additional services as well, ranging from bleach (for needle sterilization) and condom provision to HIV testing and health services to referral to drug treatment programs. There now are more than 100 needle-exchange programs operating in more than eighty cities in thirty states.[52]

Local (usually city) government has become a common forum for the struggle over how to stem HIV transmission among injection drug users and their sexual partners. These decision makers face the difficult challenge of reconciling an abstinence mandate from above with the de facto reality of harm reduction-based exchanges being conducted on the ground, often with high disregard for the legal implications. Across the nation, city governments have been forced to grapple with the problems of drug use and the questions of what message to send to their citizenry, and how to send it. The answers have varied enormously, from crackdowns on needle exchangers and clients who are regarded as flouting the law by possessing illegal syringes to toleration (official or otherwise) of activist-run programs to outright appropriation or development of such programs with official city sponsorship. These decisions are always made within the context of local politics; as with the issue of AIDS education and condom distribution in the schools, the power of community and coalition-building among proponents of abstinence or harm reduction methods have been crucial in determining the direction of these decisions.

In examining how the policy struggle over needle exchange plays out at the local level, I focus once again on New York City, which is home to a high proportion of the nation's injection drug users. Stephen Joseph, the city's commissioner of public health from 1986 to 1990, provides some sense of the magnitude of the transmission problem that the city experienced during the early years of the epidemic:

> HIV infection spread like wildfire through New York City's 200,000 heroin users, from 9 percent of infected intravenous drug users in 1978, to 28 percent by 1980, to 50 percent or more by 1982. Again, as with homosexual men, the virus had ample time to seed this population long before AIDS was recognized. In addition, infection was transmitted from male IV drug users to their female partners, both through shared drug injection and sexual intercourse. Of all New York women diagnosed with AIDS in the first five years of the epidemic, about two-thirds were infected through their own use of intravenous drugs, and about one-third through a sexual partner.[53]

Joseph was forced to confront the issue of needle exchange literally from his first hour in office, when he was asked about his position on the issue at a press conference following his swearing-in. He followed up his initial response—"Anything that might help in the AIDS epidemic should be considered"[54]—with requests for support for a pilot program from Mayor Koch, the state health department, and various law enforcement officials. At that time, New York was one of eleven states (plus the District of Columbia) where possession of needles and syringes was legally restricted. Support from the mayor and the health department was lukewarm; from law enforcement, it was nonexistent.

The debate unleashed by Joseph's requests almost immediately took on racial overtones. From the start, many African-American politicians and community leaders claimed that the program was being aimed especially at African-American drug addicts and was, in the words of City Councilman Hilton Clark, "Genocide, pure and simple."[55] The city's special narcotics prosecutor, Sterling Johnson, said the plan was like "having city-run shooting galleries," and police commissioner Ben Ward, debating Joseph in an open forum before a largely African-American audience in Brooklyn, challenged him with the question, "If you want to do needle exchange, why don't you go to Scarsdale and do it there?"[56]

The whole issue essentially stalemated; Joseph, together with a cadre of (mostly white) health professionals and AIDS activists, declared that some type of harm reduction intervention was essential at this point, and law enforcement officials—together with a powerfully united leadership of the African-American community gathered from religious, political, and treatment-based circles—arguing that needle exchange was a cheap buy-out to the much larger problem of drug use in the city. New York City's largest weekly newspaper serving the African-American community, the *Amsterdam News*, listed a veritable who's who of prominent figures who were opposed to the needle-exchange proposal: Dr. James Surtis, head of Harlem Hospital's psychiatric unit; Dr. Phyllis Harridan-Ross, director of Metropolitan Hospital's community mental health program; Dr. Beny Prim, a well-known figure in the war against drugs and director of one the nation's largest treatment programs; the Black and Hispanic Caucus of the City Council; New York City's entire congressional delegation, including Charles Rangel, head of the House Select Committee on Drug and Substance Abuse; and the New York City Black Commission on AIDS.[57]

In an unprinted response, Joseph retaliated with his own high-level list of supporters for needle exchange, including the Surgeon General; the National Academy of Sciences/IOM Task Force on AIDS; the American Public Health Association (APHA); the New York County Medical Society; the World Health Organization (WHO); and the New York State Committee of Methadone Program Administrators.[58]

While the search for ideological allies continued, policy stagnated until a small community-based organization forced the issue. The Association for Drug Abuse Prevention and Treatment (ADAPT) had been formed in the 1970s to agitate for more treatment slots in the city's drug rehabilitation centers. The group nearly died a quiet death in the early 1980s but was reorganized in 1985 to address the problem of AIDS.[59] Equipped with a tiny budget ($1,500 in 1985), ADAPT was particularly involved with direct outreach, which was conducted by board members and volunteers who distributed bleach kits and condoms and worked to get addicts into methadone treatment programs. This last activity was crucial because, absent intervention from ADAPT, the typical waiting period for such a program was six to nine months.

By 1988 ADAPT had grown and legitimized in the eyes of addicts who appreciated the organization's willingness to go to places where addicts were using (most notably, shooting galleries) to provide them with bleach and condoms. It also was recognized by the New York State AIDS Institute, which provided grant money after two other nonprofits, the Community Service Society and the New York Foundation, had helped ADAPT to become a more formalized organization.[60] Although the group transformed itself outwardly, its close affinities with its clients were confirmed when Yolando Serrano, ADAPT's president, announced that the group was willing to face prosecution and lose its financial support and tax-exempt status in order to begin distributing clean needles.[61]

The debates get a bit fuzzy at this point, depending on who is telling the story. Health Commissioner Joseph claimed that he was able to dissuade Serrano from going forward with her plan, but a different source claims that ADAPT was temporarily closed and was not reimbursed for city-related expenditures for three months.[62] Either way, ADAPT's civil disobedience had an important outcome. It brought the state—in the form of then-governor Cuomo and his health commissioner, David Axelrod—back into the debate; this time they were willing to endorse a needle exchange pilot.

Resistance from the African-American community continued, as exemplified by a front-page editorial in the *Amsterdam News* on November 5, 1988—two days before the pilot program was to begin. The editorial, titled "Koch Must Resign: Koch's Needle Exchange Program," read, in part:

> What Koch is saying is this: Your clergy doesn't matter. Your politicians don't matter. Your medical community sucks wind. Your community leaders are cowards, and you Blacks and Latinos are dumb as hell. I will do precisely what I want 'cause I am the mayor.[63]

Given the extreme opposition and the constraints on the program's design, it is hardly surprising that the program did not get off to a roaring start. The number of prospective participants had dropped to 200 and the number of sites for exchange had dropped down to one—and this site was in a particularly problematic location in lower Manhattan, near City Hall, the police department, and the criminal court. Only two addicts showed up the first day, although the program eventually grew to encompass several hundred participants. Ultimately, however, the program was shut down for good when Koch's successor, David Dinkins, made good on a campaign promise to get rid of the program shortly after taking office.

By this point, however, several activist groups were operating their own needle-exchange programs throughout the city. The successful use of the necessity defense by activists in 1991[64] encouraged other underground groups, and by the early 1990s several activist programs—including the Lower Eastside Needle Exchange Program, the Bronx-Harlem Needle Exchange Program, and Saint Ann's Corner for Harm Reduction—were supplementing the work of ACT UP.

The role of ADAPT and ACT UP and the individual leadership of people such as Serrano in promoting a harm reduction strategy and forcing action by city government through civil disobedience is typical of needle-exchange programs around the country. Most have been initiated by a charismatic leader or a small and committed organization, often with tacit approval of local officials. One of the oldest needle-exchange programs in the country was begun in 1988 in Tacoma, Washington, by Dave Purchase, a drug counselor with twenty years of experience. One of the most studied needle exchanges is operated by the city of New Haven, Connecticut, with ongoing evaluation provided by Yale University. Yet here, too, needle exchange was initiated by two groups of activists: the AIDS Brigade and AIDS Community Educators (ACES). In Boston, ACT UP (and, at times, the AIDS Brigade) operated needle exchanges for at least five years prior to the city's approval of a pilot needle program (the contract for which was then awarded, in part, to ACT UP).

One of the most important factors determining how smoothly these harm reduction strategies have been implemented, at least initially, was the ethnic makeup of the target population. Generally speaking, much of the initial resistance has arisen in cities with large minority populations, particularly when the message for needle exchange has come from white municipal health officials or community activists from white, usually gay-based, organizations.

The panel discussion mentioned at the beginning of this chapter, "The Impact of Syringe Exchange on Communities of Color," was the most well-attended, and most volatile, event at the Third Annual North American Syringe Exchange Convention in 1993. This discussion served mainly to provide voice to the ideas and objections of abstinence proponents within communities of color to the work of harm reductionists who had come to the conference.

For some people, the harm reduction message was tainted because of the messenger. Gregory Davis drew a picture of needle exchange as one more program forced on the minority community from outside:

> I am one who is not in support of needle exchange because of the way it was brought to us. I deal with men in this city, and a lot of women but mainly mostly men, and one of the things that I have found out is that in order for us to really be empowered we have to write our own script because the script that was written for us is a script that was designed to fail. What has happened in every place that I am aware of in this country [is that] a pilot program occurred in a community of color. We have always been the last to know, the last to get treated, but the first to be experimented with. And I have a hard time with that.[65]

Another participant, Ellarwee Gadsden, executive director for Women First, drew an analogy to methadone treatment to express grave doubts about the limits of harm reduction approaches and the level of commitment that could be counted on in sustaining them:

> I remember how we were going to be saved by methadone. I remember how methadone and counseling were going to be linked. We were going to rescue addicts, and we were going to rescue the inner cities from crime.... Has anybody seen heroin addicts lately? When was the last time you saw methadone and counseling? When money is withdrawn, the methadone stays, the counseling goes.... What I'm hearing is a promise. We will have needle exchange and we will have counseling. The year 2000: Picture the year 2000. You will walk into a clinic, and there's a dispensing machine. In that machine are condoms and needles. That's my problem.[66]

Of course, like many other policymakers dealing with the epidemic, some leaders of the African-American community have changed their positions as new information and ideas have become available. An important turnaround in the case of New York City occurred in 1992 when Mayor Dinkins, who had suspended the city's needle-exchange program, announced that he would not block privately funded programs. This change of heart has been credited to the mayor's examination of the New Haven program, which was begun under that city's first black mayor, John Daniels.[67]

Privately funded needle exchanges continued in New York City during the administration of Rudy Giuliani, the Republican successor to Democrats Koch and Dinkins. There is palpable tension, however, between the city government and such programs. In 1998, AIDS activist groups accused Giuliani of purposely suppressing a report of his own Office of AIDS Policy Coordination. The report, which called for expansion of the city's needle-exchange programs and argued that thousands of infections could be prevented and millions of Medicaid dollars saved, was prepared in June 1997. Giuliani denied activists' claims that his office stonewalled the report to avoid controversy during his reelection campaign, although six months after the report was written he had told the *Daily News* that he still had not read it.[68]

Despite the ongoing tension between harm reduction proponents and the zero-tolerance stance of the mayor, those who favor clean needle availability got a boost from the state of New York on May 5, 2000. After eleven years of failed attempts, Assemblyman Richard Gottfried, a Democrat from Manhattan, prevailed in his attempts to legalize the sale of over-the-counter syringes. The law, which went into effect on January 1, 2001, was passed with little fanfare and no organized opposition. The crucial turnaround in opinion has been credited to information about the Connecticut experience, where needle sharing was cut in half and HIV infections fell by a third following that state's 1992 needle sale legalization.[69]

The stop-and-start policy choices of New York City have been imitated in many other cities. Needle exchange is a powerful symbol within the AIDS community and beyond. To supporters of a zero-tolerance policy on drugs, it represents capitulation. To community leaders who are worried about the larger problems created by drug addiction, it is a Band-Aid. Some harm reductionists regard it as a symbol of hope, others as a representation of pragmatism. As affected communities continue to struggle to insert their own interpretations of this controversial policy, it is difficult to envision a national consensus emerging.

As with the controversies over HIV transmission prevention among teenagers, conflicts over needle-exchange programs point out the hollowness of public policy models that envision professional government bureaucracies objectively examining the scientific evidence and drawing the "best" conclusion. Public officials, elected and unelected, are human and are caught up in the same the personal passions, morals, and values as ordinary citizens. They are constrained not only by their own moral beliefs and values but also by the sentiments of people in the communities they seek to serve, often even when they disagree with those sentiments. The belief that there are "objective" answers to the problem of HIV transmission among injecting drug users is as flawed as the belief that there can be objective policy answers to questions surrounding abortion, gun control, and a host of other policy controversies.

The Delicate Balance between Privacy and Intervention

The needle exchange and school-based AIDS prevention cases I have examined have shown several strong contrasts between the harm reduction and abstinence approaches. The abstinence approach tells people at risk to discontinue certain behaviors; the harm reduction approach says only to minimize the risky aspects of those behaviors. Traditionally, abstinence approaches have tended to promote traditional moral values by eliminating certain behaviors.[70] Harm reduction approaches, on the other hand, attempt to refrain from passing moral judgment on risk behaviors. There is an additional, usually unspoken, difference that tends to divide the two approaches. This division has to do with what the two sides regard as the appropriate role of the state in behavior change. For most proponents of the abstinence model, it is appropriate for the state to mandate (or, in some cases, ban) certain behaviors. Risk reductionists, on the other hand, believe that individual decisions and behaviors should be voluntary. The disagreement over mandatory versus voluntary AIDS prevention measures is the fundamental divide in the final prevention policy area I examine: mandatory HIV testing of newborns.

The struggle over whether to implement mandatory testing of newborns has been emotional, complicated, and divisive. As with many other AIDS policy areas, unlikely political coalitions have developed around the issues, and some positions have changed as information about HIV and its treatment have evolved over time. And, like many other AIDS policy areas, the conflicts over testing of newborns have taken place at the local and national levels, with results at the different levels affecting each other as they have unfolded.

Although there have always been calls by a handful of conservative politicians and religious leaders to institute large-scale mandatory HIV testing schemes in the United States, such ideas have been largely discredited by AIDS activists, as well as in the minds of most of the general public. There have been a few cases, however, in which that general rule against mandatory testing has been more broadly called into question; pregnant women and their infant children have constituted one such case.

The path toward mandatory testing for newborns began with an unlikely proponent. In January 1993, New York Assemblywoman Nettie Mayersohn, a liberal Democrat, met with the New York State Medical Society. The medical society told her about a large (forty-four–state) surveillance study being conducted by the CDC. The goal of the study was to determine the prevalence of HIV among newborns, so it was conducted as a "blind" study. That is, it was being conducted so that all newborns were being tested for HIV but no one knew which babies tested positive; only the overall incidence of positive tests was reported. From the CDC (and activist) perspective, this approach was reasonable: It provided valuable information about the number of babies born with antibodies to HIV without violating anyone's privacy. From the perspective of the state medical society and Mayersohn, however, this strategy made no sense: How could crucial information about a newborn's HIV status be kept from her doctor and her own parents?

Mayersohn wasted little time in responding to this new information. In March 1993 she introduced legislation in the New York Assembly mandating that mothers must be informed if their newborns tested positive for HIV. The legislation set off a firestorm of opposition. The coalition of organizations that opposed the bill included activist AIDS organizations such as ACT UP and more mainstream AIDS organizations such as GMHC, as well as civil liberties groups such as the ACLU and proponents of women's rights such as the National Organization for Women (NOW).

It also included a large number of groups that might be considered less predictable, including the League of Women Voters, the American Red Cross, and the March of Dimes.

Opponents to Mayersohn's bill have had a host of arguments to support their position. One of the most difficult things about testing babies for HIV is that by nature it is a means of testing mothers as well. If a baby tests positive for HIV antibodies, it automatically means that the baby's mother is HIV-infected. Ironically, it does not necessarily mean that the baby is infected. We now know that a majority of babies who test positive to HIV after birth are showing only that they have *antibodies* to the virus, which is not the same as having been infected. Thus, many opponents of "baby AIDS" measures oppose them precisely because they regard them as a mandatory test-by-proxy of women who have given birth. They also fear that women who know their babies will be tested will not seek medical help with their deliveries and that women who learn their HIV status without being prepared may not be able to cope with the information (or may have partners who would react negatively or even violently as a result).

For many opponents there also is the question of why this particular group has been singled out for testing. For supporters of newborn testing, the answer is obvious: because babies cannot protect themselves and therefore are reliant on their mother's knowledge for their health and well-being. To opponents, however, it is the mothers who are vulnerable, in a political sense. Noting that privacy protection has always been a hallmark of AIDS activism, opponents question whether mandatory measures would have been adopted if the target population were different. As Theresa McGovern, executive director of the HIV Law Project (which provides free legal services to poor HIV-positive women), put it, "I should have seen that this would be the first population where confidentiality protections would slip away."[71]

As strongly as the opposition to Mayersohn's bill felt, the appeal to proponents was equally heartfelt. To them, AIDS activists and civil libertarians were giving priority to the privacy of the mother at the expense of the health of the child. Proponents argued that information about the HIV status of an infant is crucial in providing appropriate medical care, such as drugs that can prevent newborns from developing the type of pneumonia that is common among people with AIDS. They feared that the voluntary approach that already was in place was leaving some women unwilling to find out about their baby's or their own HIV status; they felt that, as Mayersohn herself said,

> The opposition never understood that women cannot afford the luxury of avoiding bad news. Women must know their medical condition so they can make important healthcare decisions for themselves and their babies; they must know so they can avoid spreading the disease to others; they must know so they can make decisions on future pregnancies; and they must know so they can make arrangements for the care of their children when they, themselves, can no longer care for them.[72]

As the two sides staked out their claims, the findings of an important study added fuel to the fire. On February 21, 1994, two institutes within NIH announced the preliminary results of a large clinical trial—AIDS Clinical Trial Group Protocol 076 (ACTG 076)—that had been running since April 1991. The trial examined the effects of giving pregnant women the antiviral drug AZT during pregnancy and labor and following up with six weeks of AZT treatment to infants after birth. The study found that AZT treatment lowered the incidence of HIV transmission 67.5 percent (from 25.5 percent to 8.3 percent). Although everyone agreed that this finding was good news, it was interpreted differently by the two sides of the debate. Opponents of mandatory infant testing argued that the trial results made it all the more important that pregnant women be counseled to agree to voluntary testing while they were pregnant and that mandatory testing would divert resources and motivation from that goal. In fact, one of the groups that took this line of reasoning was the Medical Society of the State of New York. By June 1994, the very group that initially had alerted Mayersohn to the infant testing issue and had "strongly endorsed" it had withdrawn that support in favor of strictly voluntary testing.[73] On the other side, proponents of newborn testing argued that the numbers of women who might agree to voluntary testing actually would increase if women knew that their babies would be tested as a matter of course. Given that they would find out their HIV status after the baby was born anyway, they reasoned, why not find out in time to be able to participate in a positive medical intervention?

On May 26, 1994, Representative Gary Ackerman, a liberal Democrat from Queens and friend of Assemblywoman Mayersohn, introduced a bill in the U.S. House of Representatives that was similar to the one Mayersohn had introduced in the New York State Assembly. The bill was referred first to the House Committee on Energy and Commerce and then to its Subcommittee on Health and Environment, but no further action was taken. When the 103rd Congress expired at the end of 1994, Ackerman's bill—like all bills that were still in the process between introduction and passage into law—was formally dead. He reintroduced the bill in the 104th Congress, on March 22, 1995. Again it was sent to the same committee and subcommittee, but no other formal action was taken.

The lack of action on Ackerman's bill hid several tangible responses to it, however. On the national level, the Clinton administration announced that it was calling off the CDC's seven-year surveillance program of HIV infection among infants—the existence of which had impelled Mayersohn to introduce her original bill. Although the CDC denied that the suspension was politically motivated, Ackerman and proponents of infant testing strongly believed that the move was made in response to the proposed legislation (if the "blinded" study ceases to exist, there is nothing left to "unblind").[74] Although at the national level Ackerman's bill arguably resulted in the discontinuation of the CDC's surveillance study, at the state level it was used as a reason for killing Mayersohn's bill. As the session drew to a close, the Speaker of the New York State Assembly, Sheldon Silver, argued that it would be better to wait for a response to the Ackerman bill because national legislation would supersede anything at the state level.[75] As with the CDC study discontinuation, proponents of baby testing were skeptical.

The next attempt to legislate mandatory testing for infants involved an extremely unlikely political duo: the liberal Ackerman paired with conservative Republican physician Tom Coburn of Oklahoma. Coburn routinely tested his own pregnant patients for HIV and strongly believed that testing the babies of women who did not know their HIV status made sense. He also was a member of the House Commerce Committee as well as its Health and Environment Subcommittee. These committees constituted the point of original consideration for Ackerman's baby testing bill and another extremely important piece of AIDS legislation: the Ryan White CARE Act (see chapter 5). When the House Commerce Committee held its markup (a procedure in which a committee or subcommittee meets to go over a bill and literally "mark it up" with amendments) on the Ryan White bill, Coburn offered the infant testing bill as an amendment. When longtime committee member Henry Waxman (D-Calif.) requested that he withdraw the amendment and instead work with Waxman to develop a compromise testing solution, however, Coburn agreed.

The resulting Waxman-Coburn compromise that was passed as part of the House version of the Ryan White CARE Act provided that grants would be provided to states that implemented infant testing. The compromise essentially delayed the issue, however, and offered the potential of derailing it entirely. Under the compromise, states would not have to implement testing for two years from the passage of the Act. At that time, the Secretary of HHS would be directed to make a determination about whether newborn HIV testing had become a "routine practice." If (and only if) the secretary's determination was that testing had become routine, states would have two choices: to mandate the testing or to show that the HIV status of 95 percent of newborns in the state already is known (which would signal that an extremely high proportion of mothers were agreeing to voluntary testing).

As is often the case, although both the House and the Senate passed the Ryan White CARE Act, they amended it in different ways during the process. When this happens, the bill is sent to a conference committee, whose job is to reconcile the differing versions. Waxman and Coburn, as well as eight other members of the House and Senate, served on the conference committee, and the resulting House/Senate compromise on the baby testing portion of the bill was complicated and conditional. Roughly speaking, it had four parts. First, within 120 days states had to adopt CDC guidelines on counseling and voluntary testing for women, and they had to determine the state's rate of mother-to-child AIDS (or HIV) transmission. Second, approximately two years after implementing CDC guidelines each state had to show either a 50 percent reduction in perinatal (mother-to-child) AIDS (or HIV) cases compared to 1993 or that at least 95 percent of women who had received prenatal care had been tested for HIV. Third, if states failed to meet either of the two foregoing criteria, they would have 18 months to meet one of the criteria or begin mandatory testing of newborns whose mothers' status is unknown. Fourth, all of these conditions would hold true only if the Secretary of HHS were to determine that testing has become a routine medical practice.

Despite its complexity, the baby testing measures, and the larger Ryan White Act Amendments that contained it, were signed into law on May 20, 1996, by President Clinton. The complicated provisions for implementing the baby testing programs never went into effect, however. In 1996 the American Medical Association reversed its previous position and, in a narrow vote, endorsed mandatory testing of *both* pregnant women and their babies,[76] and in 1998 a congressionally mandated study by the IOM recommended that pregnant women be tested for HIV as a part of routine care.[77] Yet HHS secretary Shalala seemed to be reluctant to issue the determination that the Ryan White Act had legislated. Finally, in January 2000, she concluded that testing of pregnant women and newborns for HIV has *not* become a routine practice. Because all of the complicated procedures of the compromise CARE Act were contingent on the secretary's determination that testing had become routine, this conclusion meant that none of them would take effect. States no longer had the mandate to do mandatory testing or reach the criteria for success in voluntary testing that the Ryan White Act had outlined.

The issue was raised at the national level again in 2000. The Ryan White CARE Act, like many major pieces of legislation, requires reauthorization on a specified schedule. The Act was first passed in 1990, was reauthorized again in 1995 (though the process took so long it actually finished in 1996), and was up for consideration again in 2000. In the 2000 reauthorization the baby testing issue again was enormously controversial and resulted in a decision to use financial incentives to encourage states to set up mandatory testing programs for all newborns or for newborns whose mothers have unknown HIV status.

Although opponents of mandatory newborn testing have been successful in preventing federal legislation requiring such testing, they lost in the initial battleground state of New York. In 1996, Governor George Pataki signed Public Health Law (PHL) 2500-f, mandating that doctors test all newborns and inform mothers of the results.

The New York State program has been implemented in two phases; the first phase began on February 1, 1997. During this phase, all babies were tested for HIV, and the results were given to the baby's mother and doctor. Although the first phase was very successful in notifying mothers of their babies' and their own HIV status and referring them to appropriate care, the program suffered from a weakness that had been predicted by its opponents: HIV test results often were not available for two weeks—precluding timely administration of AZT.[78]

This issue was addressed in the second phase of the program, which was initiated on August 1, 1999. Based on the medical finding that AZT can reduce the transmission of AIDS even if it is given during the first 48 hours after birth,[79] in this phase expedited HIV testing was ordered in all cases in which an HIV test result from prenatal care is not available.[80] In February 2000, the director of the New York AIDS Institute, Guthrie Birkhead, wrote that the rates of prenatal care were being examined, and there was no evidence that rates of participation in prenatal care had declined—as many opponents of baby testing had feared.[81] The program also appeared to be having a very high success rate in identifying HIV-exposed births and referring HIV-positive mothers and babies for early diagnosis and treatment. In a letter to Dr. Peter Van Dyke, associate administrator for the Maternal and Child Health Bureau within HHS, Coburn quoted the director of the New York AIDS Institute in claiming that universal testing had identified all HIV-exposed births in that state and facilitated 98 percent of them in getting appropriate medical treatment.[82] These high figures were consistent with a statement from Mayersohn's office dated September 5, 2001. Using numbers from the New York Health Department's AIDS Institute, Mayersohn noted that "of the 4,022 HIV-exposed infants identified under the law since 1997, 99.4 percent have had follow up medical care" and "women are being tested in higher numbers, more women are receiving prenatal care, and lives are being saved."[83]

As with most of the policy areas I discuss in this book, the issue of mandatory testing for infants is far from resolved. Information from the New York program, together with that of Connecticut (which followed New York in passing its own law in October 1999), will be closely examined by both sides. New York State's experience has not quelled the fears of most testing opponents, who continue to worry that testing of newborns will open a wedge for other forms of mandatory testing and infringe on the rights of expectant mothers. Conversely, proponents have continued their fight to see mandatory testing implemented at the national level, as exemplified by Ackerman's introduction of the Newborn Infant HIV Notification Act once again in May 2000. (Although Coburn signed on as a cosponsor, he retired at the conclusion of the 107th Congress, so he will not be on hand in the House to press the measure in the future.)

The Struggle Continues

Although almost all policy areas have financial dimensions, the divisions over policies designed to meet the challenge of HIV/AIDS prevention are *not* primarily financial. Although both sides sometimes resort to financial rhetoric, arguing that *their* side has the more cost-effective approach, the more important factor is a struggle over underlying values. What is really at stake is how the challenge of HIV/AIDS prevention should be defined, and what values to follow when pursuing a plan of action. Which is more important: information and choices for young people or the supervision rights of their parents? Is it better to help drug users mitigate the negative consequences of their actions or insist that they refrain from drug use? Is it more important to respect the privacy rights of mothers or to know the HIV-status of their children? These are tough choices, and they do not have financial solutions. They will continue to be debated as long as there is diversity of opinion in the larger society.

CHAPTER 5

A New Means of Providing for the Sick:
The Ryan White CARE Act

In 1990 the U.S. Congress did something new. For the first time ever, it provided money to help people who were bound together not by age or income or disability but by a virus. The Ryan White CARE Act provided funding for the needs of people with AIDS and HIV infection. Less than ten years later, as lobbyists gathered to push for its second reauthorization (the first was in 1996), disagreements had popped up everywhere. States were arguing that they needed some of the money that was being specifically targeted to cities. Activists were accusing AIDS organizations of spending too much on salaries and not enough on clients. Gay-based organizations and minority-based organizations in the same cities had fought over who should get the bigger share of the money allotted to those cities. Scandals were surfacing about the misuse or outright embezzlement of funds. Renegade AIDS denialist organizations were siding with conservative Republicans that too much money was being spent, period. And AIDS organizations in the cities of Los Angeles and San Francisco were flinging mud at each other with abandon. What had happened?

At the heart of the controversy is the classic issue of all government distribution policies. When governments distribute something people want, it is entirely predictable that more than one group will make claims on what is being distributed. And no matter what formula is used for making distributive decisions, some groups feel short-changed and attempt to create a different distribution plan. There is an additional problem that also is not unique to AIDS. As organizations are awarded contracts and are paid by the government to provide services, like all organizations they seek to maintain their size and, if possible, grow more. This can happen only if they are able to maintain or, better yet, increase their share of the government funding. Putting together these two types of groups (those that want to change the funding formulas and those that want to maintain them) is an instant recipe for conflict.

The original decisions about how to provide for people with AIDS arose from a broad definition of how HIV affects the people it infects. People with AIDS and HIV infection have certain medical needs, but that is only the beginning of the story. When people are sick, they need more than just medical treatment. Illness can render us incapable of going to work, and that can cause us to lose not only our income but also our health insurance and our homes. When we are sick we may be unable to conduct many ordinary activities, such as feeding ourselves, cleaning and maintaining our homes, and transporting ourselves wherever we need to go. For people at the lowest economic levels of society, such as homeless people and those living in areas with few public services, these activities already are enormously challenging; being sick only makes them more so.

When illness is widespread, it affects the needs of the community as well. As people take on the problems of their families, friends, and neighbors, they too feel the stress and anxiety created by illness. They also may need to find out how to keep themselves well and how to prevent further transmission of the illness that is taxing the community. Thus, services such as educational programs, testing and counseling, and support groups may be created to help meet community needs as well as individual needs. Especially in the early days of the AIDS epidemic, community-based organizations were called on to help with all of these problems—to help take care of people who were ill as well as administer to the "worried well." The work was expensive, time-consuming, and draining, and AIDS service organizations began to ask local government, and later the federal government, for help.

The U.S. Congress reacted to these calls for help by passing the Ryan White CARE Act, which was created to secure special funds for medical and social services for people with, or affected by, AIDS or HIV. Of course, Congress passes funding bills all the time. One of the special and unprecedented attributes of this specific bill, however, was that, for the first time, funding was to go to people solely on the basis of their infection with or risk status for a *specific* disease. This point was not lost on president George Bush, who signed the bill reluctantly, warning that "the bill's narrow approach, dealing with a specific disease, sets a dangerous precedent, inviting treatment of other diseases through similar arrangements."[1]

On the surface, there were many signs that the new policies created by the Ryan White CARE Act were uncontroversial. After all, the bill's chief cosponsors in the Senate were conservative Republican senator Orrin Hatch and liberal Democrat Ted Kennedy. It was named after one of the most famous and respected people who has died of AIDS, teenager Ryan White. And it passed both houses of Congress by overwhelming votes: 95 to 4 in the Senate and 408 to 14 in the House of Representatives.

Yet the bill's seemingly uncontroversial passage covers a multitude of policy struggles underneath. The Ryan White CARE Act delivers ever-increasing resources (that is, money) to help pay for a variety of activities that are designed to help people infected with and affected by HIV and AIDS. It is only natural that there will be disagreements over how those resources will be divided. How do we know who qualifies as "infected with or affected by"? Which services are needed most by these people? Are the problems worse among certain groups or in certain geographic areas? Who gets to decide? All of these questions, and a great many more, were decided when the Act was passed in 1990, and not everyone was thrilled with the initial answers. In 1996 and again in 2000, when the Act was reauthorized for the first and second times, these issues were reopened and debated, as people with many different visions came together to try to decide the best way to distribute the money.

The Original Recipe: The 1990 Ryan White CARE Act

One feature of the AIDS epidemic in the United States is that it was first recognized in cities—particularly Los Angeles, New York City, and San Francisco. The earliest community-based responses, which involved mostly AIDS service organizations run by and for the gay community, also sprang up in cities, to meet the needs of people who were coming down with the mysterious and deadly new syndrome. It is not surprising, therefore, that when activists began to push for funds to deal with the epidemic, they billed it as an urban disaster. Recall, for instance, the full name of the Act itself: the Ryan White Comprehensive AIDS *Resource Emergency* Act.

The Act's name was politically significant in another sense as well. The people who were pulling for this legislation were well aware of the criticism by President Bush and other critics that the bill would set a precedent for spending. Some of the services that would be funded would include categories that verged dangerously close to the dreaded label of welfare spending (or entitlement spending, in academic lingo)—including medical care, case management, and food provision. Therefore proponents went out of their way to distance themselves from being seen as advocates of another welfare program and argued instead that the Act was an important form of disaster relief.

One group that pushed for the Ryan White CARE Act was the National Organizations Responding to AIDS (NORA). NORA is a group convened by the AIDS Action Council, which is the major Washington, D.C., lobbying group for AIDS-related organizations. NORA is an organization of organizations, including member groups such as the PTA, the American Red Cross, and a host of other national groups with at least a peripheral interest in AIDS policies. According to a letter that NORA wrote to members of the House of Representatives about the proposed Ryan White Act, "The bill deals with the health disaster brought to a few American cities. Like Hurricane Hugo and the San Francisco earthquake, the human tragedy of AIDS in a number of disproportionately impacted cities requires federal assistance."[2] Almost five years later, when the Act was up for reauthorization, the same argument was made again. For example, in 1995 Mark Barnes of the AIDS Action Council claimed—about as directly as a person could—that "the Ryan White CARE Act is not a welfare program, and it is not an entitlement."[3]

Another political strategy that was employed in getting the Ryan White CARE Act passed was the deliberate selective framing of who would and should benefit from the new legislation. Indeed, although the gay community contributed enormous levels of support to lobbyists and organizations that pushed Congress to support the Act, that involvement would be difficult to discover by listening to the speeches of House and Senate members. Supporters of the Ryan White CARE Act often relied on stories about individual people with AIDS in making their case for the urgency of the legislation. According to one study, nineteen such stories were told in all, but the demographic characteristics of the people of those stories are very telling. Of the nineteen stories, six were about Ryan White himself, five were about infants or children, three were about women, two were about recipients of tainted blood or blood products, and one gave no demographic description. Thus, although the gay community was putting enormous energy into the issue, only one of the nineteen stories featured a gay man (who also was described as an injection drug user) to support the idea that the Ryan White CARE Act was desperately needed.[4]

So what did the Ryan White CARE Act do? As passed in 1990, the Act was composed of four parts, or titles. The first and largest part of the four (imaginatively called Title I) was the "disaster relief" part of the bill. It provided for direct aid to the metropolitan areas hardest hit by the epidemic. During the first fiscal year (1991) of the Act, sixteen cities qualified as eligible metropolitan areas (EMAs). To qualify for this designation, a metropolitan area had to have a minimum cumulative caseload of 2,000 or at least 0.0025 percent of its population by June 3, 1990. More metropolitan areas were added to the list later as they hit the qualifying minimums: Two more qualified in 1992, seven qualified in 1993, and another seventeen qualified in 1994 and 1995 combined. As of 1999 there were fifty-one qualifying EMAs.[5] To meet the standard, some regions were defined quite broadly. The EMA of Boston, for example, included most of Massachusetts as well as three counties in southern New Hampshire![6]

Once an EMA qualified as part of Title I, the amount of funding it received also was based on the cumulative caseloads. That is, the more cumulative cases of AIDS since 1981 or the more cumulative cases per thousand, the more money the EMA was entitled to receive. Predictably, the epicenters of the epidemic, New York City and San Francisco, received—and continue to receive— the largest amounts of Title I funding.

The EMA's mayor (or chief elected officials, if the EMA was an urban county) was to create a new organization (or designate an existing one) to serve as an HIV Health Services Planning Council (HHSPC). The job of this new official-sounding group was to look at what was being done already and what needs were unmet, to come up with a plan for the best delivery of services, and to decide whether funds were being efficiently allocated. In other words, the HHSPCs would be in charge. They would get to decide the all-important question in politics: who gets what. Therefore, the creators of the Ryan White legislation took pains to require that the makeup of the HHSPCs would be inclusive. Indeed, according to directions from the Health Resources and Services Administration (HRSA)—the government agency in charge of carrying out the Ryan White CARE Act—HHSPCs had to have representation from at least eleven different types of groups, including a gamut of different types of professionals, local leaders, and affected communities. Yet these precautionary measures were not enough, in the eyes of some people, to guarantee that the HHSPCs were completely fair and representative.

Title II of the Ryan White CARE Act was created to ensure that each of the fifty states got some money to deal with the epidemic. Each state was guaranteed a minimum grant of $100,000; funding went up from there on the basis of states' cumulative caseloads and fiscal capacity, as determined by average per capita income. Thus, states that had experienced more overall AIDS cases and had more lower-income people could expect larger grants than states that did not. Each state had to use at least part of its Title II grant to come up with entities known as "HIV care consortia" that would provide "a comprehensive continuum of care to individuals with HIV disease and their families."[7] Each state consortium was supposed to come up with a series of services that would best serve HIV-positive people and their families in that particular region or state. Each state could decide how many consortia to establish; the number ranged from only one in some states to a high of forty-four in California.[8]

Beyond establishing the care consortia, there were special rules on how a state could spend its Title II money. The money could be spent on home- and community-based care services but not inpatient services (that is, regular hospital care). It could be spent to help a private individual keep up with private health insurance payments but could not be spent to replace state Medicaid funding. It also could be spent on medical treatment designed to "prolong life or prevent serious deterioration of health." Title II also singled out infants, children, women, and families by requiring that states spend at least 15 percent of Title II grant money specifically for these groups. As initially enacted, HRSA also had the power to set aside 10 percent of total Title II funds for Special Projects of National Significance (SPNS); this provision was changed in 1996 to make funding of SPNS a separate program under the Act.

In contrast to Title I and II funds, Title III funds bypassed cities and states entirely. Instead, Title III was used to fund individual programs from public and private nonprofit organizations (including migrant, community, and homeless health centers, as well as hemophilia treatment centers) that were already dealing with at-risk populations. The purpose of Title III was to facilitate early intervention in people who were at risk for and infected with HIV by increasing funding for testing, transmission prevention programs, and medical and social services.

Compared to the other titles, Title IV fared rather poorly with regard to allotment of money. The purpose of this title was to provide family-centered, community-based services to children, youth, and women living with HIV. It was not funded at all during fiscal years 1991 to 1993. Later, funding from this title was used to fund a variety of projects, including programs designed to decrease HIV transmission from pregnant mothers to their babies and projects that aimed at helping HIV-positive adolescents.

Although the Ryan White CARE Act was a major departure for Congress in many ways, in others the Act has been typical of the way the federal government spends money. As with most spending bills, *authorization* and *appropriations* for the Act have looked very different. When Congress passes an authorization bill, such as the original Ryan White CARE Act of 1990 or the reauthorizations of 1996 and 2000, it is creating the *possibility* of spending whatever amount it authorizes in the legislation. In other words, it sets a ceiling above which spending cannot go. In August 1990 both the House and the Senate agreed to pass the Ryan White CARE Act with an authorization of $875 million for the first year it would go into effect. In October of that same year, however, when the two sides had to agree on the actual *appropriation* (that is, how much the government would actually spend), the number was less than a quarter of the original authorization—only $221 million.

Another way in which the Ryan White CARE Act is a typical product of Washington is its growth. Although activists were disappointed in the discrepancy between the original authorization and the first year appropriation, funding for the Act, like most government programs, has grown over time. The number of EMAs covered by Title I has grown from sixteen in 1991 to fifty-one in 1999. The total amount of annual spending under Title I also has grown: from roughly $86 million in the first year of funding under the Act (fiscal year 1991) to approximately $485 million in fiscal year 1999. Congress also has inserted new programs that are now an important part of Title II funding. Perhaps the most significant and fastest growing are the ADAPs. Although states were always directed to use a portion of Title II money to provide assistance for drug therapies, in recent years this program has become extremely significant. As combination therapies have become increasingly common (and increasingly expensive), states have experienced dramatic increases in their ADAP spending.[9]

Although the major growth in Ryan White CARE Act funding has benefited many different organizations and constituencies within the AIDS community, disputes over how the money should be spent and whether limitations should be placed on it have grown over time. These disputes have resurfaced most obviously during the debates over major reauthorizations, first in the period from 1995 to 1996 and again in 2000. In the remainder of this chapter I examine these two reauthorization periods and discuss some of the struggles and debates that occurred among AIDS-affected communities that the reauthorizations brought to light.

What's Fair When People Are Dying?

One of the major strengths of the complicated Ryan White CARE Act was that, for the most part, it funneled money to the state, city, and community levels. Proponents of the Act point out that localized control has allowed policymakers to deal with the epidemic flexibly. They could respond to the needs of local HIV-positive and at-risk populations, which vary tremendously in demographic characteristics and risk behaviors from one state or EMA to the next. What might be useful, for instance, for a city where the primary risk behavior is injection drug use would be very different from an area where most of the cases were among men having sex with men.

In many places, however, the assumption that local control means fair distribution has been strongly challenged. The first such challenge occurred, ironically, in spite of unprecedented strong rules about inclusion in the HHSPCs (which administered Title I) and consortia (which administered Title II). Recall that the HHPSCs were mandated to have representation from at least eleven different types of groups. According to critics in at least some cities, however, the reality was that the first community-based groups to be established in the area sometimes had the most control. Many of these groups arose within the community where HIV/AIDS was recognized first: the predominantly white gay and lesbian community. When other communities, particularly minority communities, began to recognize the increasing incidence of HIV within their populations, minority leaders sought to push new organizations into an already well-stocked pool of groups that were not looking for new competition. In *The Gravest Show on Earth*, author Elinor Burkett quotes Tim Palmer, a gay man who has worked in the AIDS service industry in the Northeast for more than a decade:

> What has happened is that gay white men in cities like San Francisco and New York were the first people at the table.... Once they got control over the table, they shut it off, both locally and nationally. Sure, they let a few others come and sit down—but not so many that they can make independent decisions.[10]

The Ryan White CARE Act had a dual mission: efficiency and inclusion. But what if these two goals come into conflict? Should the contract go to the organization that has been around the longest and "knows the ropes" or the group that best represents the population at risk or infected? Although the demographics of the epidemic were shifting over time, control of Ryan White CARE Act funding in many areas did not necessarily reflect those shifts.

In Washington, D.C., for example, the clash centered on the Whitman-Walker Clinic. Originally founded as a gay and lesbian health center, in the early days of AIDS organizing Whitman-Walker filled a crucial void of service provision. This same early work put it in a powerful strategic position for distributing funds when they started flowing into the District of Columbia through the Ryan White CARE Act. One result was that "by 1993 more than 60 percent of Washington's AIDS cases were among blacks, but only 20 percent of the CARE Act money was being funneled through black community-based organizations."[11]

The "got there first" advantage seemed to have been duplicated in Boston as well. There, the director of the Latino Health Institute took issue with many of the principles used by the Boston AIDS Planning Council for deciding who should receive Ryan White CARE Act funding. In a letter to leaders of the Council he questioned why it gave priority to "existing organizations over new organizations" and "agencies that can demonstrate existing linkages to other services in the continuum."[12] In his view these principles were inherently discriminatory because "they have the direct effect of excluding non-dominant communities from fair competition based on present need, rather than history."[13]

In Dallas, the same dynamics (giving priority to whatever organizations "got there first") created the opposite problem: Gay-based organizations were the ones excluded. As a consequence of a conservative and homophobic political culture, the city had a history predating passage of the Ryan White CARE Act of giving priority to the (mainly heterosexual) organization AIDS Arms at the expense of the (mainly gay) AIDS Resource Center (ARC). When Dallas was named one of the original sixteen Title I EMAs and money began to flow in, by statutory definition Dallas County Judge Lee F. Jackson was the chief executive officer of the EMA. He took pains to minimize the number of openly gay appointees, but he placed several AIDS ARMS representatives on the Planning Council. As of 1997, gay men held only one-third of the seats in the Planning Council for the Dallas EMA, although at least 75 percent of the caseload over the prior two years was gay men (in previous years that proportion was even higher).[14]

Still another variation of the "getting there first" problem revolves around the value of national name recognition. In *The Boundaries of Blackness* Cathy Cohen writes about the fact that funders of legislation such as the Ryan White CARE Act are more likely to "give funding, especially among marginal groups, to those organizations with national name recognition, like the Urban League or the NAACP."[15] She also notes, however, that those granting the money often do not closely examine whether these groups have the ability to directly target the groups within the black community that need it most. Moreover, these groups often coordinate the services of others, rather than actually providing services themselves. In New York City, for instance, Cohen notes that the New York Urban League runs the Central Harlem HIV Network. The money comes from Ryan White CARE Act funding allocated through the city Planning Committee, although the Network does not provide any direct client services; it merely coordinates the services of other groups.[16]

While the battle over inclusion was fought at the local level, a second struggle within the "AIDS establishment" was waged in Washington. Again, the issue was fairness, but the scope had shifted. Instead of arguing over which segment of a community was most deserving of money, the conflict was over *which communities* deserved the most money. This struggle started when the executive director of the AIDS Resource Center of Wisconsin, Douglas Nelson, compared the funding levels for services being provided in Milwaukee to those in San Francisco. He had expected that they wouldn't be exactly the same, but he was shocked at just how different the numbers were. What Nelson calculated was that Milwaukee was getting about $1,000 per person living with AIDS while San Francisco was getting more than $6,000. Nelson also discovered the keys to the difference; those same keys were found by GAO, which conducted a study on the same issue.[17]

There were two causes for the difference. The first was that Title I funding was based on cumulative caseloads. In other words, the caseload was counted as all people who had been diagnosed with AIDS thus far. The two most heavily funded cities in the country, New York and San Francisco, had the two highest cumulative caseloads. The difference in per-person expenditures that Nelson found between those cities and Milwaukee came from the fact that approximately 60 percent of the individuals counted in the cumulative figures of the first two cities had died, yet they were still counted in the official formula.

The disparity was made even larger by a second problem: double counting. The backers of the original Ryan White CARE Act had argued that it should serve as disaster relief for cities and a source of money for planning and service coordination for the states. Consequently, caseloads were counted separately for Titles I and II. Therefore, people with AIDS in the cities were being double-counted—once for the cities and again for the states—even though the states often funneled some of their Title II money back to the cities to help pay for AIDS services. People with AIDS in states that did not have a qualifying EMA were counted once, however— for the Title II money only.

As with many government programs, the Ryan White CARE Act led to the creation of groups of people with interests in keeping the program alive. Thus, the quest for continuing money through reauthorization of the Act saw some new groups that hadn't been around for the 1990 legislation. The original major lobbying group for AIDS-related programs from the government, the AIDS Action Council, was now joined by a host of new organizations. The new, expanded coalition included Cities Advocating Emergency AIDS Relief (CAEAR), which was concerned mainly with Title I; the National Alliance of State and Territorial AIDS Directors, which had come into being because of (and was interested in preserving and increasing) Title II; the National Ryan White Title III(b) Coalition, which represented the 136 nationwide health centers funded under that title; and the AIDS Policy Center for Children, Youth, and Families, which represented projects funded under Title IV.

Nelson met in Washington, D.C., with this enlarged group of organizations to present his arguments for a new funding formula.

To Nelson's surprise, CAEAR (the group that had convened the meeting) did not share his interest in a funding adjustment. Viewing the Washington AIDS establishment as hostile to his goal of reforming the formula, Nelson then created his own group. The new coalition, the Campaign for Fairness, was composed mainly of community-based health and service providers whose cities did not qualify for Title I money but got CARE money through Title II state allotments. Armed with evidence from the GAO report, the Campaign for Fairness convinced the Senate Labor and Human Resources Committee, which was responsible for writing the reauthorization legislation, to reconsider the funding formulas. At the same time, the Campaign worked with the AIDS Action Council, which reluctantly agreed to support changes in the formula—with one condition: a "hold harmless" provision under which allocations to the cities in the greatest danger of losing funds—San Francisco and New York—could decrease by no more than 7.5 percent, and the decrease would be spread over seven years.[18] Although Nelson saw the issue strictly in terms of dollars per patient, representatives of Title I EMAs pointed out that cuts created by reallocation would be felt most strongly by already-underserved communities of color and other disadvantaged groups.

The AIDS Action Council's conditional position failed to satisfy the needs and desires of all of its constituencies, however. On June 13, 1995, the San Francisco AIDS Foundation, one of the country's largest and oldest AIDS groups, wrote a letter to the Council denouncing the Council for "robbing Peter to pay Paul and calling it 'equity.'"[19]

Another issue that surfaced during the 1995 reauthorization focused not on what *areas* deserved money but on whether the money should come with strings attached. There has always been a difference of opinion between liberals and conservatives over the appropriate role of privacy protection when dealing with HIV prevention (see chapter 4). In 1995, one aspect of this debate was played out when Republican Representative (and medical doctor) Tom Coburn attempted during committee deliberation of the bill to insert a provision for mandatory testing of infants. Representative Henry Waxman, a liberal Democrat, asked him to withdraw the amendment and work out a compromise to be passed in its place. That compromise (which I discuss in detail in chapter 4) delayed the issue of testing for two years, until the Secretary of HHS determined whether newborn HIV testing had become a "routine practice." The compromise was then replaced in conference committee by a more complicated procedure that provided for several possible state actions regarding infant testing, all contingent on a determination by the Secretary of HHS.

In the end, the reauthorization formally became Public Law 104-146 on May 20, 1996. The struggle over reauthorization revealed several things. On one hand, it demonstrated the political strength and momentum that the AIDS movement had gathered during the decade. Although Republicans had replaced Democrats as the majority party in Congress in 1994, the Ryan White CARE Act reauthorization enjoyed the same high levels of congressional support it had received in 1990. At the same time, however, the reauthorization revealed fault lines that were beginning to develop *within* the AIDS movement. In 1990 the goal had been to convince Congress of the need to provide money for the needs of people affected by a single disease. In 1995 the key issue had become how that money (and, preferably, much more money) could be handed out most fairly and efficiently. As members of the AIDS movement have discovered, achievement of the first objective has been much simpler than the second.

Third Round: The Questions Just Get Tougher

Like the 1996 reauthorization, the second reauthorization in 2000 was fraught with controversy. In 1996 the major battles had been over the best way to count AIDS caseloads and which potential funding beneficiaries might best serve clients; in 2000 these questions were supplemented with other distribution questions. One tough issue involved disparities between urban and rural areas. When the Act was first passed it was billed as emergency relief for cities besieged by an extraordinary health care disaster. Ten years later, rural health delivery systems were arguing that they also needed more money to minister to the needs of people infected and affected by HIV.

Although the issue of disparities between rural and urban areas ultimately were addressed by changes in the 2000 reauthorization, it proved to be far less controversial than another geographic issue that had come up in 1996: differences in Title I funding for cities. In 1996 the issue had been difficult; in 2000 it only got more so. In 1996 the compromise had been to make sure that no city would ever lose any more than 7.5 percent of its funding and that such a loss, if it happened, would be spread over seven years. By the 2000 authorization, however, several conservative Republicans (whose party now controlled Congress) were ready to challenge that compromise. As House Commerce Committee Chair Thomas Bliley wrote in a letter to the California congressional delegation on the differences in levels of funding per person with AIDS in different cities, "This unfair disparity is a lingering artifact of pre-1995 policies embedded in the Ryan White CARE Act that paid for treatment based on the number of AIDS patients, living and dead, who were diagnosed in any given EMA. The era of paying for the treatment of the long dead is long over."[20]

In 1996 the "hold harmless" provision had benefited four EMAs: Houston, Jersey City, New York, and San Francisco. By 1999, however, San Francisco was the only one still benefiting. Not surprisingly, San Francisco—especially its largest community-based AIDS service organization, the San Francisco AIDS Foundation—was thrown into a defensive posture. Proponents for San Francisco, such as Representative Nancy Pelosi, argued that any major shift to bring San Francisco's per patient funding in line with other areas would be unfair. Part of the reason the number of AIDS cases in San Francisco was reduced, Pelosi noted, was that the city had been so successful in helping people that there were more people living with HIV (but still requiring expensive medical therapies) and fewer with the full-blown AIDS diagnosis that was the basis for funding. As Pelosi argued, "We can't be penalized for intervening earlier and prolonging life."[21]

The situation may have been especially bitter because another California city, Los Angeles, entered the fray and soon joined the more outspoken elements that wanted a more drastic reapportionment than the 1996 compromise. Pelosi referred to this development as "unfortunate";[22] the Internet was soon buzzing with a leaked e-mail that said a lot more than that. The e-mail, which made the rounds of electronic lists of AIDS activists around the country and was covered by the *Bay Area Reporter*, was written by an employee of the San Francisco AIDS Foundation to a staffer of the Office of AIDS Programs and Policy for the Los Angeles County Department of Health Services. The May 9, 2000, message accused the director of that office, Charles Henry, of being a liar and "nothing but a pimp."[23] Although the San Francisco AIDS Foundation's Pat Christen apologized for her employee's words after they had been brought to her attention by Henry's boss, the incident highlighted the level of contention over the funding disparity.

A very different controversy, larger than the Ryan White CARE Act but strongly related to it, involved differing views of the concept of need itself. When the epidemic began, early AIDS service organizations—almost all rooted in the gay communities of urban areas—had addressed the problems created by AIDS by providing a wide array of services to infected people and the larger community. These services included health care or linkages to health care, case management, social support systems such as buddy programs for infected people, and hotlines and prevention programs for the larger community. Many of these services came to be supported by funds from the Ryan White CARE Act, in addition to community fundraising. By the time of the 2000 reauthorization, however, the picture of need had changed somewhat. For several reasons, including the advent of HAART regimens (i.e., the "cocktail") I discuss in chapter 2, many of the people traditionally served by the programs offered by many AIDS service organizations had less need for those services. The need for supplemental funding for AIDS drugs through the ADAP programs funded in Title II skyrocketed, however. Through new therapies, these people were showing fewer and fewer signs of being sick. Many were able to go back to work and maintain their homes and daily activities without the help of volunteer and professional services. This is not to say that the services offered by AIDS service organizations were now obsolete, nor does it deny the fact that AIDS has increasingly become a disease of lower-income people with greater need for certain services. These changes do suggest a shift, however, in the overall dimensions of need; as drug therapies become increasingly effective in controlling the effects of HIV, access to these therapies becomes a major priority. To the extent that access to drug therapies is successfully expanded, the other services of AIDS organizations should become less necessary.

This changing dynamic of need has contributed to an internal debate within the AIDS community. In this debate, the lines are drawn primarily between the (mostly volunteer) radical activist groups, such as various ACT UP chapters, and the (mostly professional) AIDS service organizations benefiting from Ryan White CARE Act funding. From the activist perspective, the service organizations are in danger of losing the idealism with which they were founded. The activists worry that the AIDS service organizations that had begun out of a desperate need for someone to address the enormous unmet needs created by a terrible new illness had evolved into stereotypical self-perpetuating bureaucracies. Ryan White CARE Act funding, in the activists' eyes, had made the situation worse. With money comes the ability to pay salaries, turning volunteer positions into paid ones. With money comes programs, and with programs come the need to show continuous (and, ideally, growing) need for whatever the programs provide. Activists began to throw around the term "AIDS industry" to describe the groups and individuals that were most concerned with maintaining funding streams, even when conditions might necessitate a new focus on other issues.

This internal conflict put reform-minded activists in an awkward position. On one hand, they were interested in rooting out corruption and guaranteeing that Ryan White CARE Act funding was flowing as directly as possible to the clients who needed it most. On the other hand, they were acutely aware that exposure of such misconduct brought them into common cause with groups and individuals who were interested in criticizing beneficiaries of the Act for a very different reason. For these critics, the real goal was to rechannel Ryan White CARE Act funds away from AIDS spending altogether. One of the most notorious critics was long-time foe Jesse Helms, who had unsuccessfully attempted to block the 1996 reauthorization by arguing that Congress was "falling all over itself to do what the homosexual lobby is almost hysterically demanding" and that homosexual behavior is "incredibly offensive and revolting.[24] Other congressional adversaries, as well as conservative interest groups such as the Family Research Council, agreed with Helms's long-held sentiment that AIDS funding was too high, especially compared to funding for other diseases.

Other groups—most importantly the renegade AIDS denialist group ACT UP San Francisco—used the debate as an opportunity to make the claim that because AIDS did not exist, Ryan White CARE Act funding was a scam. Thus, activists for reform found themselves weighing their words and actions carefully in an attempt to argue that funding had to continue, although reforms were equally necessary.

Thus, for the third time, the Ryan White CARE Act represented more than a way for Congress to give money to sick people and those who cared for them. This time it served as a forum over whether more attention should be paid to rural health and service delivery and whether there should be disparities in funding among cities receiving grants. Furthermore, professionals working with AIDS and HIV found themselves on the defensive, forced to prove that the money they asked for was still going to desperately needed services, not for the perpetuation of bloated bureaucracies.

As with the 1996 reauthorization, in 2000 Congress asked the GAO to conduct a study, and the results of this study helped set the tone for the new round of debates. The GAO was asked to focus its study on several specific questions: who was benefiting from the Ryan White CARE Act, demographically speaking; what types of expenses the Act was paying for; whether the current approach to funding in the Act was advantageous; whether Ryan White CARE Act services were reaching rural areas; and whether the salaries of administrators of AIDS service organizations were in line with those of administrators at similar nonprofit organizations.[25]

The GAO report findings were quite positive. The report found that the Ryan White CARE Act was serving typically underserved groups, such as poor and uninsured people. In fact, according to the GAO, African Americans, Hispanics, and women were being served "in higher proportions than their representation in the AIDS population."[26] The report also found that people with HIV and AIDS in rural areas were getting Ryan White CARE Act drug assistance in proportion to their incidence in rural areas. The report further noted that other services were reaching rural residents as well, although "data do not exist to show where the individuals receive the services."[27] Finally, the report found that median salaries in AIDS organizations receiving Ryan White CARE Act funds generally were comparable to those in similar nonprofits.[28]

These generally positive findings from the GAO did not match the perceptions of several critics of the Act's beneficiaries, however. As is often the case when activists attempt to bring attention to an issue, local activists chose to focus on several important symbolic cases to demonstrate their argument that the AIDS bureaucracy had become removed from the people it should be serving. One lightning rod for criticism was San Francisco AIDS Foundation Executive Director Pat Christen. In addition to being embroiled in the continuing controversy from the 1996 reauthorization over funding formulas for Title I EMAs, the San Francisco organization came under fire for the salary it provided Christen. According to a 1999 *San Francisco Chronicle* story on the subject, Christen was being paid $175,000 annually, which several activists, particularly those from all-volunteer organizations, considered unacceptably high. As Jeff Getty, community activist and member of ACT UP/Golden Gate noted, "Listen, I think Pat would be great running Chevron, but she's not the right person to be running an AIDS nonprofit that was founded to be caring, accountable, and community-oriented." Christen retaliated that her detractors were sexist, claiming, "I think some of my critics are not comfortable with a woman in a position of leadership making the money that I do."[29] One of Christen's strongest critics, the *Bay Area Reporter*, editorialized on May 25, 2000, not only that Christen's salary was "bloated" but also that the Foundation itself had become "unaccountable and inaccessible."[30]

Despite the GAO report's finding that administrative salaries for Ryan White-funded AIDS service organizations were roughly in line with those of similar nonprofits, examples like the Christen case caused at least some volunteer activists to work together with unusual legislative partners. ACT UP chapters—particularly ACT UP/DC, which had taken the lead in pursuing perceived instances of unaccountability within the AIDS industry—met with former foe Tom Coburn on several accountability issues. Coburn requested the GAO report that specifically examined the salary issue, partially in response to activist demands. His office was sympathetic to a host of proposals that activists led by ACT UP/DC suggested as ways to increase accountability. Among the proposals were a requirement that at least one-third of the Title I planning councils be composed of "nonaligned" consumers who were not employees, board members, or consultants of groups getting the money; "sunshine rules" guaranteeing that Title I planning council meetings and their proceedings be open to the public; auditing of organizations receiving Ryan White CARE Act funds; and a salary cap for top AIDS administrators that would limit salaries to the level of the chief elected official (usually a mayor) of the area where the administrator lives.

A second example of excess highlighted by several AIDS activists occurred as the Senate was considering the Ryan White CARE Act's 2000 reauthorization. In this case the spotlight was turned not on a single individual but on a whole group— namely, AIDS service and treatment providers receiving money under Title III of the Act. The providers were on the hot seat for attending a conference, the Third Annual Clinical Update on HIV, sponsored by the HIV/AIDS Bureau of the HRSA. What annoyed activists was not the conference itself—similar meetings had been held in New Orleans and Tucson—but the conference locale and funding. The conference was held at a beach resort on St. Thomas in the U.S. Virgin Islands; U.S. Delegate Donna Christian-Christensen had played a key role in increasing Title III funding to allow for such conference attendance and in bringing the conference to the area she represented.

Defenders of the conference, including Christian-Christensen (who is a medical doctor) and the San Francisco AIDS Foundation's Ernest Hopkins, argued that the conference was a chance for mainlanders to be exposed to health care delivery in a developing area.[31] Wayne Turner, speaking for ACT UP/DC, found such arguments unpersuasive, however, pointing out that the conference was by invitation only, local people with AIDS had not been invited, and conference activities were scheduled on the grounds of the resort hotel.[32] According to the *Virgin Islands Daily News*, on the second day of the conference Christian-Christensen had issued a statement inviting local physicians to attend the meeting for free. Yet members of the Community Planning Group, leaders of the local HIV/AIDS treatment community, "didn't know a thing about it," according to board member Dr. Henry Karlin.[33]

Christen's salary and the Virgin Islands conference may be unacceptable by some standards, but it is hard to label them outright scandals. That distinction belongs to the now-defunct San Juan AIDS Institute in Puerto Rico. San Juan had been one of the original sixteen EMAs and as such had qualified for Title I money from the beginning. As early as 1993 a Puerto Rican legislator, David Rodriguez Noriega, wrote to HHS Secretary Donna Shalala alleging corruption on the part of the San Juan AIDS Institute; he received a form letter reply for his trouble.

The allegations of corruption did not formally bear fruit until 1999, when more than $2 million dollars, much of it Ryan White CARE Act Title I money, were found to have been embezzled from the San Juan AIDS Institute. In a sensational trial that galvanized the attention of Puerto Rico (although it went largely unreported in the mainland United States), lead defendant Yamil Kouri and several of his associates at Advanced Community Health Services, which ran the AIDS Institute, were found guilty of stealing federal funds, obstructing justice, and money laundering. Among the testimony were allegations that $250,000 of the embezzled money had found its way into the political campaigns of the governor of Puerto Rico, Pedro Rosello, who had been director of the Health Department of San Juan and had selected the AIDS Institute directors who were convicted in the trial.[34] Although Rosello, as well as several other politicians, denied knowledge that their campaigns had accepted money from the AIDS Institute, members of the local Puerto Rican activist organization, AIDS Patients for Sane Policies, joined with ACT UP/DC to demand a full audit of Puerto Rico's federally subsidized AIDS activities.

Although the Puerto Rico scandal was the largest misuse of funds in dollar amounts, activists have highlighted smaller improprieties on the mainland as well. Around the same time that a second San Juan trial was beginning (June 2000), the *Dallas Morning News* reported that the FBI was investigating a nonprofit south Dallas AIDS clinic. Although the story reported that the clinic had significantly improved its operations since October 1998, when county auditors began to question its practices, the FBI investigation is ongoing. Among the allegations are charges that the clinic had rung up $60,000 worth of psychic hotline calls, that public funds had been spent on Neiman Marcus shopping sprees, that expensive AIDS drugs were unaccounted for, and that the clinic may have submitted bills for treatment of patients who never existed.[35]

The Representative Coburn–ACT UP/DC coalition went to work on the issues of salaries, secrecy, and misallocations as a package. A press release from Coburn's office discussing the call for the GAO report also mentioned not only the Puerto Rico scandal but also that the head of the North Carolina-based Drug and AIDS Prevention Among African-Americans had written himself checks and "kept books that were unauditable." In the letter requesting the GAO audit sent by Coburn along with majority leader Dick Armey and Commerce Committee chair Thomas Bliley, question number five (of ten questions transmitted) was, "Is there any evidence of abuses or misuses of federal AIDS funds?" Although the GAO did not answer the question in its report, the issue was taken up with great energy by Coburn's office and ACT UP/DC. Coburn's office sent out several press releases and letters seeking audits and questioning procedures; ACT UP/DC posted many of these documents, together with its own commentaries, on the ACT UP/DC website and activist electronic lists. Coburn also was able, at ACT UP/DC's request, to bring in Jose Colon, president of AIDS Patients for Sane Policies (the watchdog group that had formed in reaction to the Puerto Rico scandals), as a key witness in July 11, 2000, hearings before the Health and Environment Subcommittee of the House Commerce Committee.

While the reformist coalition was working on these accountability issues, the renegade denialist group ACT UP/San Francisco attempted to go one step further and use the allegations of misuse to support its larger claims that AIDS is not caused by HIV and is not a threat. With much fanfare, ACT UP/San Francisco began to publicly urge Congress to cut funds for the Ryan White CARE Act. In May 2000 the group sent 450 information packets to Capitol Hill urging that all federal funding for AIDS be cut, and in June it followed up with a full-page ad in the Capitol Hill newspaper *Roll Call* (other Washington papers refused to run it) listing examples of misallocated funds and headlined with the exhortation to "Pull the Plug on AID$ Fraud!"[36] Although the group's antics did not have the desired effect of decreasing AIDS funding, it did provoke a reaction from other ACT UP organizations—particularly ACT UP/New York and ACT UP-Philadelphia, which released a joint press release and wrote a joint letter to Congress disavowing any connection with the denialist group.

Although the Coburn–ACT UP/DC coalition worked together on accountability issues, it had areas of significant disagreement. Representative Coburn also viewed the 2000 authorization as a vehicle for implementing the mandatory testing and partner notification policies that had failed in the 1990 legislation and the 1996 reauthorization. As chapter 4 details, these mandatory policies are strongly opposed by almost all AIDS activists. In 2000, however, other elements of the political landscape had changed in Coburn's favor. Chief among these changes was the fact that there appeared to be strong support for the idea of mandatory testing of infants from several quarters. The IOM had done a study on the issue and recommended that a national policy of HIV testing (and partner notification) be adopted as a routine part of prenatal care. As Coburn pointed out when he testified before a Senate Committee on the issue in July 2000, the AMA, the American College of Obstetricians and Gynecologists, and the American Academy of Pediatrics all endorsed the position as well.[37]

The 2000 reauthorization passed near the end of the 106th Congress and, like its predecessors, vote tallies for the bill made it appear uncontroversial. It received 411 votes in the House and passed the Senate by a unanimous voice vote. In reality, however, several compromises had been required to get the measure through. AIDS activists lost the fight to cap the salaries of AIDS organization administrators, but they did prevail on several other accountability reforms. The 2000 version of the Ryan White CARE Act carried the requirement that a third of the Title I planning council members be unaligned consumers and helped make those consumers' voices stronger by providing training for new members to help them fully participate. In the new version, planning councils would be required to figure out how much of the Ryan White CARE Act money was being used to provide overhead and how much was actually going to services. In addition, the federal government each year would now audit random samples of CARE Act recipients and subcontractors.

Coburn in large part lost his fight to reapportion money away from San Francisco when a compromise was brokered to limit San Francisco's funding cut to 15 percent—about $7.5 million over five years, rather than the original $40 million over five years he had proposed. He prevailed in other areas, however. Rural areas received an increase in funding, and the reauthorization definitively moved into the areas of testing and partner notification that had been held at bay during the 1990 and 1996 rounds.

In the area of infant testing, Title II now authorizes a new appropriation of $30 million targeted primarily at states that set up mandatory infant testing for all newborns or for newborns whose mothers have unknown HIV status. There also is a requirement for a second IOM study that will determine the incidence of HIV in babies with mothers of unknown HIV status, barriers to routine testing, and recommendations for reducing perinatal transmission. Title II also provides for a new grant program for partner notification for states that do contract tracing and provide that information to the CDC.

Conclusion

The perennial issues of distribution—who is deserving of government resources, how should those resources be fairly distributed, and what strings should be attached—have been answered, at least until the next five-year increment. The patterns of the answers (as well as the arguments themselves) since the original passage in 1990 offer us some insights, however, into the larger AIDS policy landscape. The original law was a reflection of its time. When it was drafted, the only approved antiretroviral drug on the market was AZT. Almost all of the country's AIDS service organizations were still identified with the gay community and were highly dependent on volunteers performing a host of support functions, and the incidence of HIV/AIDS was highly concentrated in a few urban areas. The intersection between gay politics and AIDS politics that this situation created also guaranteed that privacy concerns—always a major item on the gay political agenda—would be translated into AIDS policy as well. So it is not surprising that the 1990 Ryan White CARE Act was targeted toward providing financial relief for large cities and that gay-identified AIDS service organizations would become major political actors in the distribution process. It also is not surprising that the Act's funds would be dedicated to supporting a wide range of social services, including case management, rather than being targeted primarily to drug procurement. Equally unremarkable, in this context, is the absence of mandatory testing and partner notification in the original law.

As the decade progressed, however, the general political landscape and circumstances regarding HIV/AIDS in the United States changed. In 1994 Republicans became the majority party in Congress, vowing to downsize government and reintroduce more conservative social policy. On the AIDS front, important strides were made in the treatment of HIV infection that promised significant health gains, at increasing financial costs. The AIDS community itself, once united in its argument that the country desperately needed to devote more resources to manifold needs of HIV-infected people and their communities, was experiencing a split. The AIDS service organizations had professionalized and become big-budget operations at the same time that many in-the-streets activists had begun to wonder if government money wouldn't be better spent directly on drugs and possibly direct financial assistance. At the same time, the demographics of HIV infection continued to shift, so that HIV disease increasingly became a problem of people of color, injection drug users, their sexual partners and families, and poor people.

In some ways, the changes in 1996 and 2000 reflect those shifts. The influx of conservative Republicans in Congress almost certainly contributed to the inclusion of partner notification and infant testing measures in the 2000 bill. Perhaps as significant was the fact that resistance toward these measures had softened, for several reasons. Some testing advocates argued that the effectiveness of the new medicines made early treatment more desirable and testing therefore more necessary. A more cynical argument of some activists was that the stakes weren't the same for gay-based organizations that in 1990 had argued against mandatory testing on behalf of their communities but did not identify as strongly with the communities that in 2000 were more likely to be the subjects of these policies. Another reflection of the changing times was the unlikely Coburn–activist coalition that brought about significant accountability changes in the 2000 law.

Just as telling as the changes that occurred in 1996 and 2000, however, are the elements of the Ryan White CARE Act that stayed the same or changed only marginally. These elements highlight several truisms in politics and policymaking. One is that it is much easier to give something to a group than it is to take it away.

A second is that the criteria for allocations are politically determined. The idea of who is "most deserving" is politically charged, with few if any objective means available to help policymakers decide. Instead, other rules of thumb become salient. How long a group has been around, how nationally well known a group is, and how well organized a group is internally don't say much about the deservingness of its members or clients. Yet with the Ryan White CARE Act, as in many other policy areas, all of these considerations have become important determinants in how resources have been allocated.

The most dramatic example of these truisms occurred in San Francisco, which managed to hang onto almost all of its funding in the face of calls for dramatic formula changes not once but twice. San Francisco has hardly been alone in the quest for funds, however. A notable feature of the Ryan White CARE Act has been its sheer growth over time—in numbers of cities qualifying for Title I, in dollar amounts for all titles of the Act, and in new programs appended to the original Act. As Americans who are concerned about the impact of HIV/AIDS in our communities, we have responded with a national policy to provide resources to address the problem. As the struggles in 1990, 1996, and 2000 all illustrate, however, there is no way to shield this Act from the contentious process that is inherent in all distribution policies.

CHAPTER 6

Us and Them: AIDS as a Foreign Policy Issue

Every two years experts from around the world convene at an international AIDS conference to present the newest information about prevention and treatment of HIV infection. The Thirteenth International AIDS Conference was held July 9–14, 2000, in Durban, South Africa, marking the first time the event was held in a developing country. The host nation had the dubious distinction of having the largest number of HIV-positive people in the world (an estimated four million), which helped to focus the world's attention for a few days on the plight of all of the nations of sub-Saharan Africa. Collectively, these countries have felt the brunt of the AIDS pandemic; although they account for only about 10 percent of the world's population, they account for approximately 70 percent of the world's HIV-infected people.

Unfortunately, much of the opportunity for focusing the spotlight on this grave international crisis was squandered by the huge amount of attention paid to a single speech—that of South African President Thabo Mbeki. By the time the conference began, Mbeki already was in disfavor with many conference attendees for his activities during the weeks prior to the conference. In addition to personally questioning the link between HIV and AIDS, he convened a panel of international experts to reexamine this issue, which the vast majority of AIDS scholars consider definitively settled. He refused to give AZT to his country's pregnant HIV-positive women to stem the transmission of HIV to their babies, citing the problems of the questionable link, the possible toxicity of AZT, and the expense. Then he used his opening remarks to conference attendees to argue that extreme poverty, rather than AIDS, was the leading killer in sub-Saharan Africa. On December 14, 2001, Mbeki's government lost on this issue when the South African high court ruled in favor of AIDS activists and pediatricians who brought a class action suit against the government arguing that by providing treatment only at pilot programs, the government was discriminating against mothers who gave birth at other hospitals.[1]

Whereas Mbeki's speech was widely covered, a second major speech received much less attention. That speech was made by Edwin Cameron, who delivered the first Jonathan Mann Memorial Lecture. Cameron, a South African High Court justice who has been open about his HIV-positive status in a country where such disclosure opens the possibility of deep discrimination, used his opportunity in the spotlight to highlight a position that activists on both sides of the Atlantic had been promoting for some time. In a stirring appeal to the world's moral conscience, he argued that we are living in an era in which complacency is comparable to supporting a system as wrong as Nazi Germany or apartheid South Africa:

> The inequities of drug access, pricing and distribution mirror
> the inequities of a world trade system that weighs the poor with

debt while privileging the wealthy with inexpensive raw materials and labour.

Those of us who live affluent lives, well-attended by medical care and treatment should not ask how Germans or white South Africans could tolerate living in proximity to moral evil. We do so ourselves today, in proximity to the impending illness and death of many millions of people with AIDS. This will happen, unless we change the present government ineptitude and corporate block-ing. Available treatments are denied to those who need them for the sake of aggregating corporate wealth for shareholders who by Africa standards are already unimaginably affluent. That cannot be right, and it cannot be allowed to happen.[2]

During the same week that Cameron spoke from the podium, his ideologi-cal allies spoke from the streets. They were led by South African activists belonging to the Treatment Action Campaign (TAC), with support from the U.S.-based Health Global Access Project (GAP). The protest against an international system of drug pricing that made AIDS drugs that are so vital for treatment in western countries totally out of reach of almost all Africans constituted one of the largest AIDS pro-tests ever. More than five thousand people—including South African religious groups, labor unions, and gay and lesbian rights groups that had all endorsed TAC—con-verged on the eve of the first day of the conference to participate in the Global March for Treatment Access.

The drama that played out in the conference rooms as well as outside in Durban is a microcosm of the struggle that is going on in the developing and devel-oped worlds. The confrontation is very uneven. One side (the world's developed coun-tries) has almost all of the resources and tools for dealing with HIV and AIDS; the other (the developing—that is to say poor—countries) has almost all (approximately 90 percent) of the actual cases. Figuring out what to do about this gap may be the most important challenge worldwide for AIDS policymakers. Because the United States is the richest and most powerful country on earth, as well as the one where HIV and AIDS were first formally discovered and have been copiously researched for the past two decades, it is, by necessity, a major player in the search for policy solutions.

The people with the most at stake in U.S. policy choices in this area mostly live outside our borders. Nevertheless, the stakes for them as well as for many actors within the United States are extraordinarily high: millions of lives hang in the balance. Thus, the final major policy issue I examine in this book is AIDS as a foreign policy issue. Because this issue involves so many people, so many problems, and so few resources (as yet, anyway), it is far more complicated than any of the other issues I have discussed in this book. In fact, it encompasses all of the other issues I have exam-ined—research, drug treatment, the blood supply, prevention efforts, and social ser-vices—but compounds them with the additional complications of an international setting, profound cultural differences, and extreme poverty.

To get a handle on such an immense topic, I focus on one region of the world (sub-Saharan Africa), with particular emphasis on the country of South Africa. Similarly, I examine only a few of the policy challenges that have thus far created policy struggles involving the United States. There are a great many policy players in the international arena of AIDS policymaking: governments; grassroots activist groups; nongovernmental charitable and service organizations on the national and international levels; private, for-profit groups, including national and multinational corporations; and international governmental organizations such as those sponsored by the United Nations. Again, in the interest of simplicity, I narrow the scope and focus on only a few of these groups, though in each case I examine, many more actors are involved.

The actors I focus on can be clustered in three main categories: government entities, including agencies and groups and individuals within Congress; activist organizations, particularly those belonging to the U.S. treatment access group known as Health GAP; and private, for-profit corporations, particularly those that manufacture pharmaceutical products (which are mostly multinational corporations). Because this chapter deals with how these groups and individuals act *internationally* in addition to how they interact with one another within the United States, I make reference to other actors outside our borders. These other actors include groups within foreign governments, particularly South Africa; other activist groups, such as South Africa's TAC and France's ACT UP/Paris and *Medecins San Frontieres (MSF)*/ Doctors Without Borders; and international governmental groups such as WHO.

Roughly speaking, recent U.S. foreign policy regarding AIDS in Africa has revolved around three issues. The first, a precondition in a sense for others, has been simply raising the salience of AIDS in sub-Saharan Africa as a concern worthy of attention and financial resources, and then increasing those resources. This is an enormous challenge because this area of the world traditionally has been a low priority for the United States, and it slipped even lower during the 1990s. The major U.S. government agency that handles nonmilitary foreign aid, USAID, openly states that Africa is the area of the world in greatest need of financial support. According to USAID numbers, Africa has the lowest per capita gross domestic product (GDP) ($560, compared to Asia's $730 and Latin America's $4,230), highest infant mortality rate, lowest life expectancy, and highest HIV/AIDS incidence of any region of the world. Yet in fiscal year 2001, USAID's Development Fund request to Congress was approximately $532 million. This amount is less than the amount requested for Eastern Europe and the Baltic states ($610 million) and far less than the controversial $1.6 billion military aid package President Clinton requested for the country of Colombia to further the drug war there.[3] Moreover, although the United States is the richest country on earth by far, USAID reports that by 1996 it had dropped behind France, Germany, and Japan in its level of donations to Africa.[4] Thus, activists working to procure more money for Africa were working against a trend that deemphasized the region as an area requiring U.S. attention.

The second issue (which is too multidimensional to address fully in this chapter) has revolved around the question of debt cancellation and the concurrent goal of increasing the means by which sub-Saharan nations can devote a greater proportion of their own resources to the AIDS crisis. This second issue has engendered a worldwide activist movement that is very broadly based. Proponents of debt cancellation all agree that the poorest countries of the world have been saddled with massive levels of debt—often because of political circumstances that are far beyond the control of most of the citizenry of the affected countries—that they will never be able to pay back. Furthermore, proponents argue that the cost of attempting to pay back the debt creates unacceptable societal problems because heavily indebted countries must divert money that is desperately needed for social spending on health, education, and infrastructure to payments on the interest of previous loans. Countries that cannot make their payments must apply for yet more loans to service their existing debt, and they usually are subject to requirements to institute structural adjustments—changes to the economy to privatize government-subsidized enterprises such as education and health care. Thus, either way, according to activists who want to see the debt canceled, the existence of debt is inhibiting developing countries from spending their own money to provide programs that would help these countries actually develop. Given that AIDS activists believe that many more resources need to be devoted to HIV prevention and treatment, they are in agreement with the larger movement that seeks debt cancellation and have worked in alliance with that larger movement on this issue.

Finally, there has been the issue of drug availability and pricing. This issue has generated the most explicit debate and action by actors on both sides of the policy struggle in the United States; therefore I devote the majority of my attention in this chapter to this issue. Roughly speaking, the issue has pitted activists against pharmaceutical companies, with the U.S. government playing an uncomfortable role in the middle. The struggle has been one of competing ideologies. On one hand, the pharmaceutical companies have argued that intellectual property protection is absolutely essential to innovation. Absent a guarantee of profits from a patented discovery, this side argues that companies will lose the incentive to create the products that have raised the quality of life—and provided life itself—for millions of people. On the other side, AIDS advocates and activists argue that this very profit motive is killing people. To them, the goal must be to get as many drug treatments to as many people as possible. If generic manufacturers can do that at a price that is accessible to the people who are dying, it is the obligation of others in government and the private sector to allow, and even facilitate, that process.

The U.S. government finds itself in a difficult position. Many members of Congress as well as presidential candidates (current and potential) have important stakes in the welfare of the pharmaceutical industry: It is a major contributor to congressional and presidential campaigns and a major employer in some congressional districts. Furthermore, many politicians, particularly conservative Republicans, agree with the pharmaceutical industry in principle that innovation depends on protecting intellectual property at all costs. On the other hand, others in government are less convinced of the sanctity of intellectual property, and many are personally upset by the crisis created by HIV/AIDS in the developing world. Politically speaking, however, they have little motivation to take action because the people who are suffering most from this crisis are not U.S. citizens. They do not vote here, and they are far too poor to affect campaign contributions. Thus, they must rely on the good will of politicians who are continuously pressed by their own constituencies to put a plethora of issues ahead of this one.

On an abstract level, the questions raised by HIV/AIDS as a foreign policy issue revolve around the critical policy-related concept of *membership*, which in this case usually translates into citizenship. The assumption that nation-states have different (and larger) obligations to their own citizens than to people outside their borders is so deeply ingrained in our policies that we seldom question it. Yet even if we accept this assumption, HIV/AIDS brings up questions at the margin. Do we owe *anything* to people outside our borders? Is a nation obliged at least not to make the situation worse (for example, by blocking access to affordable medication options) for people struggling in other countries? If a state has to decide between marginally raising or maintaining the well-being of its own citizens or greatly raising the well-being of people outside its borders (for example, by increasing foreign aid that will cost a few dollars per citizen but will greatly benefit people in other countries), what should it do? The vast magnitude of the human catastrophe of AIDS in developing countries and an increasing awareness in the United States of that catastrophe has brought these questions—which usually simmer quietly on the important but underemphasized back burner of development politics and policy—squarely to the fore.

A Crisis of Astounding Proportions

Before delving into the policy struggles that are being waged over AIDS in Africa, I need to sketch out a few of the dimensions of the problem itself. In a world where poor people are disproportionately suffering from HIV infection and its effects, the people of sub-Saharan Africa are bearing the worst toll of any world region. According to a Joint United Nations Programme on HIV/AIDS (UNAIDS) update released in December 2000, the proportion of adults living with HIV/AIDS in sub-Saharan Africa is eight times that of the rest of the world (a prevalence rate of 8.8 percent, compared to the 1.1 percent average worldwide). Of the 36.1 million people estimated to be living with HIV/AIDS, 25.3 million of them live in Africa south of the Sahara. Of the world's estimated 5.3 million new infections in 2000, 3.8 million—or 71 percent—occurred in sub-Saharan Africa, compared to the 45,000 new infections (less than 1 percent of worldwide new infections) in North America.[5]

The fact that the epidemic clearly is causing the most new infections, illness, and death in sub-Saharan Africa is compounded by the intense poverty of most of the people infected and affected. This combination of illness and poverty create a situation in which every aspect of the disease—from medical care to the creation of orphans through the death of parents to the challenges of implementing prevention programs—creates strains on already overtaxed systems. When parents grow sick or die, children can no longer pay their school fees and are forced out of school. When adults are sick, have to spend all their time nursing other family members, and eventually die themselves, there is no one to do even subsistence farming. Women survivors can be forced to become sex workers to support themselves and their children, thereby multiplying not only their suffering but also the spread of the virus itself. As the virus continues to spread, the already low level of educated professionals in areas such as teaching, the military, the government bureaucracy, and health care are hard hit as well. As Dr. Peter Piot, executive director of UNAIDS, explains, "HIV does to society what it does to the human body. It undermines the very institutions that are meant to defend society—its teachers, its doctors."[6] In a Pulitzer Prize–winning series titled "AIDS: The Agony of Africa," journalist Mark Shoofs provided the *Village Voice* with a compelling picture of the level of misery the virus has caused. In the eight-part series that ran November and December 1999, he details the lives of elderly grandparents with no source of income attempting to raise large numbers of orphaned grandchildren, morgues crammed beyond capacity with bodies, and people with AIDS who are so poor that starvation will surely kill them before the virus that has incapacitated them.[7]

Many analysts and activists who are concerned about the AIDS crisis in sub-Saharan Africa link it to a related problem: the region's staggering external debt. Jubilee 2000 is one of many organizations that are dedicated to resolving this problem through cancellation of the debt by the World Bank and developed nations to whom it is owed. Jubilee 2000's report, *Eye of the Needle: The African Debt Report*, offered a set of summary findings in the introduction. The summary notes that sub-Saharan Africa owes $231 billion to its creditors, which breaks down to $406 per African. Foreign aid, it reports, cannot keep pace with the debt: For every dollar received in foreign aid in 1999, the region paid back $1.51 in debt. The cost of this debt servicing translates into an enormous deficits in resources for other social spending: Sub-Saharan Africa spends more than twice as much on debt servicing as it spends on basic health care.[8] Thus, many activists argue that a crucial part of any policy dealing with HIV/AIDS in sub-Saharan Africa must be eliminating or greatly reducing the region's external debt so that national resources may be refocused on prevention, treatment, and development efforts.

Given the tremendous scope of the problem, some people might question whether *any* efforts from outside the region could help. AIDS advocates around the world believe they most assuredly could. Coping with the devastation wrought by the pandemic can be thought of as a three-pronged effort. Resources will be needed for education and prevention efforts designed to stem the tide of new infections; medical treatments to help people who already have the virus; and financial assistance to deal with the societal cost of the pandemic, including the creation of millions of orphans and the lost productivity caused by the death of so many people in their most productive years.

In one of the earliest calls for serious assistance, UNAIDS initially suggested a sum of $3 billion annually would go a long way toward alleviating the problem. Half of the money was to be used for massive prevention efforts, and the other half was to be for treatment to deal with pain relief and opportunistic infections (but not antiretroviral medications, which at that time were considered too expensive even to contemplate providing) and to help cover the costs of orphan care. In comparison to the resources and spending habits of rich nations, especially the United States, this amount is affordable. As Piot has pointed out, "This is a fraction of the $52 billion that is spent annually in the U.S. on obesity."[9] Moreover, grassroots activists on both sides of the Atlantic have successfully challenged the original assumption that antiretroviral medications are not a practical treatment option. Although the retail cost of more than $10,000 a year for the AIDS "cocktail" in the

United States clearly is prohibitive, activists have argued that other existing alternatives, such as generically manufactured cocktails that have been offered to developing countries for $500 per year (and recently even less) could put them within reach of at least some people.

Figuring in the additional costs of drastically less expensive antiretrovirals has led analysts to some new estimates that are higher than Piot's original but still within the capacity of developed countries to fund. The most famous such estimate is the $7–10 billion called for by UN Secretary General Kofi Annan for a global fund that would be used to address the problems of HIV/AIDS, malaria, and tuberculosis.

Having briefly sketched the dimensions of the HIV/AIDS crisis in sub-Saharan Africa, I turn back to the main focus of the chapter, which is to examine the policy response to this crisis by the United States. I examine the long process that was required to wrest an acknowledgment of the crisis and a financial response from the U.S. government. I also trace the evolution of the ongoing policy struggle among activists, the government, and pharmaceutical companies over how to provide medical treatment for people suffering from HIV infection. Although I introduce these two issues separately above, their actual evolution has been closely intertwined. In fact, one might argue that at times policymakers have sought to substitute one response (acknowledge the problem and give limited amounts of money) for the other (allow countries to get affordable drugs). Thus, the following discussion is similarly intertwined.

The Slow Path to Awareness

The first issue—raising the profile of HIV/AIDS—has taken two basic forms in the United States. One has been rhetorical; it is evident in debates over the level of priority given to international AIDS issues, as well as in how they are framed. The second goes beyond rhetoric and takes the form of the actual level of financial commitment given by the U.S. government. In both cases, critics of the U.S. government have regarded the U.S. response as too little, too late. The problem has been not so much lack of information as inattention to the information on hand.

The struggle over simply making AIDS in developing countries, particularly in sub-Saharan Africa, an important problem to policymakers dates at least to 1987. That was the year that CIA intelligence officer Katherine Hall and her colleague Walter Burrows began lobbying their agency for personnel and equipment to study the growth of AIDS globally. Their requests were denied, and colleagues offered opinions that reflected a very low level of concern and awareness. One suggested that the coming AIDS crisis might be a good remedy for African overpopulation, another that the deaths of officers in foreign armies from the disease would lift morale because there would be more room for advancement from underneath. Three years later, Hall and Burrows finally received the go-ahead to research Interagency Intelligence Memorandum 91-10005—a report that was released in 1991 as a classified document titled "The Global AIDS Disaster" that foretold of 45 million infections worldwide by 2000.[10] The response was underwhelming: No one asked about the document except for then-Surgeon General C. Everett Koop and a Pentagon medical unit.[11] In 1992 the CIA gave the State Department unclassified portions of its work to be released as part of a white paper. More people read it, but the level of response did not improve.

During the mid-1990s, elements of the U.S. government continued to resist acknowledging the impact the epidemic was having in developing countries. This resistance was driven by several motivations. Fear of creating a demand for services that could not be met; desire to retain control of agency budgets; and the belief that money would be better spent on other, more cost-effective measures than those addressing HIV all played into decisions by agencies such as the CDC and USAID.

At the same time, the U.S. government and its agencies were not getting a lot of pressure from activist groups to act any differently. The mid-1990s were a time of hope for the HIV-infected in the United States (see chapter 2). As the discovery of AZT gave way to the increased effectiveness of combinations of drugs, AIDS became a more readily treatable condition. The urgency in the United States turned from developing drugs to finding ways to pay for those that had been developed for all HIV-positive citizens, and the politics of AIDS advocacy adjusted itself accordingly. In 1993, for example, GMHC rebuffed a representative of ACT UP/New York who broached the problem of drugs for people with AIDS in Africa with the response that there were still people in the Bronx who couldn't get AIDS medications.[12] Some critics of the slow U.S. response to AIDS in Africa also regard racism as a motivating (though unspoken) factor. UNAIDS head Piot has been quoted as saying that "if this would have happened in the Balkans, or in Eastern Europe, or in Mexico, with white people, the reaction would have been different."[13]

The drug companies that manufacture treatments for opportunistic infections as well as the powerful new antiretroviral combination therapies exhibited a similar lack of urgency. Although the major drug companies held meetings about the subject beginning in 1991, in the early 1990s they appeared to reach consensus only on the idea that price discounts to developing countries would be a bad idea. They felt that it was up to governments to worry about distribution and accessibility problems, that AIDS drug regimens were too complicated to adapt to developing-world conditions, and that numerous other barriers existed in African countries. Given these opinions, it is hardly surprising that the talks ended altogether in 1993.[14]

Ironically, although the rise of effective and expensive combination therapies in a sense explicitly turned AIDS spending into a zero-sum game in which U.S. AIDS advocates saw money going to efforts outside the country as money that could be spent on underfunded ADAPs, these same drugs freed other activists to turn their attention to sub-Saharan Africa and other developing regions. ACT UP/New York's Eric Sawyer explains, "When you are no longer burying your friends, you have the luxury of time to try to save people in more remote areas. There is a tremendous sense of survivor guilt, which gives us inspiration to fight harder."[15]

Two other related developments of the late 1990s helped to create more favorable conditions for a new more globally oriented wave of AIDS activism. The first was the rise of a parallel movement of other activist causes that were loosely organized as a backlash against the forces of economic globalization. These activists' causes varied widely, from environmentalism to labor and human rights to debt reduction. All of these groups, however, shared a distrust for the rise of a global free market that, in their view, opened the way for the extraction of resources and cheap human labor to benefit multinational corporations at the expense of the environment and poor people worldwide. AIDS activists share many of the beliefs and goals of this larger movement and have formed alliances within it.

The second development that facilitated the activism of global AIDS activists and the antiglobalization movement was the rise of the Internet. Computer-mediated communications, including e-mail, listserves, and websites, greatly increased the level of contact and the pace of campaigns, as activists from around the world were able to organize actions in advance with allies from other continents and find out almost instantaneously how they were proceeding.

Two examples of the beneficiaries of this new technology are the U.S.-based Health GAP and the South African-based TAC. Although it is possible that both organizations could have formed and operated independently of computer technology, there is no doubt that such technology has greatly facilitated their work internally and with each other.

TAC is the older of the two groups; it was founded on December 10, 1998 (International Human Rights Day). TAC exists to raise public awareness about the affordability and accessibility of HIV/AIDS treatments—an important issue in the country with the largest total number of HIV-positive people in the world. TAC works to achieve a mass base and has been very successful in achieving alliances with other public interest organizations. The South African Council of Churches, the Congress of South African Trade Unions, the National Coalition for Gay and Lesbian Equality, and a host of other groups have endorsed it. TAC has been an extremely active participant in the policy struggle over intellectual property rights for pharmaceutical products.

TAC's U.S. ally, Health GAP, is a collection of activist and advocacy organizations and individuals. Founded in March 1999 by New York City physician Alan Berkman, it brings together consumer advocacy groups, including two groups founded by Ralph Nader (Consumer Project on Technology and Essential Action); activist groups such as ACT UP/Philadelphia and ACT UP/New York; self-empowerment AIDS advocates such as John James, editor of *AIDS Treatment News*; and human rights groups such as the International Gay and Lesbian Human Rights Commission. Health GAP also has worked in alliance with other international organizations, including *MSF*/Doctors Without Borders, ACT UP/Paris, Network of People Living with HIV/AIDS in Thailand, and several other grassroots AIDS organizations in developing countries. Together with TAC and other allied organizations, Health GAP has launched the Global Treatment Action Campaign (GTAC), which is committed to creating first and third world activist partnerships to achieve access to medications for HIV and other diseases. Although these groups' main goal relates more clearly to the second major issue of this chapter—providing affordable treatments to HIV-positive people in sub-Saharan Africa—their actions have provided greater visibility to the struggle for achieving recognition and funding for the AIDS crises in Africa as well.

If Compulsory Licensing Is Theft, Is AIDS Profiteering Murder?[16]

After the inactivity that marked the 1980s and most of the 1990s, activity around AIDS policy in Africa increased dramatically from 1999 to 2001. Much of the activity stemmed from the 1997 decision of the South African government to amend its Medicines and Related Substance Act of 1965 with a new provision referred to as Article 15(C). The amendment was passed over the objections of U.S. pharmaceutical companies operating in Africa and U.S. Ambassador James Joseph. The drug companies and Joseph appeared before the South African parliament to testify against the amendment. The problem with the amendment, from opponents' perspectives, is that it appears to allow the South African government to resort to practices known as compulsory licensing and parallel importing. Essentially, compulsory licensing allows a government to permit a third party to manufacture a product without the permission of the party that holds the product's patent. Compulsory licensing could occur, for example, if a country authorized its own factory to produce a specific drug without the permission of the company that owns the patent for that drug. Parallel importing occurs when someone other than the authorized distributor is permitted to import a product. Parallel importing usually occurs because of differences in prices in different countries and thus might be described as "global bargain shopping." The problem, according to the pharmaceutical companies, is that the practice amounts to theft—or something very close to it. They believe that if a company holds the patents on specific drugs, the company alone should be able to sell the product, and it alone should be able to decide at what price to sell it for different markets.

The United States and South Africa are member nations of the World Trade Organization (WTO). The WTO exists to facilitate international trade by reducing trade barriers between countries and resolving trade disputes. To belong to the WTO, member states must agree to abide by its rules, one of which is an agreement on trade-related aspects of intellectual property (TRIPS). The WTO allows compulsory licensing and parallel importing, subject to specific rules and safeguards.

The initial struggle over the South African law revolved around a reading of WTO rules. The pharmaceutical lobby and the U.S. government maintained that the TRIPS agreement prohibited South Africa's new law. South Africa, together with several other developing countries and AIDS activists inside and outside the United States, maintained that the law was in compliance with the TRIPS agreement and that the United States was in essence demanding "TRIPS-plus"—a level of compliance even higher than the standard set by the WTO.

That the issue was taken seriously by the U.S. government is documented by a U.S. State Department report summarizing efforts to convince South Africa to change its policy:

> All relevant agencies of the U.S. Government—the Department of
> State together with the Department of Commerce, its U.S. Patent
> and Trademark Office (USPTO), the Office of the United States
> Trade Representative (USTR), the National Security Council (NSC)

and the Office of the Vice President (OVP)—have been engaged in an assiduous, concerted campaign to persuade the Government of South Africa (SAG) to withdraw or modify the provisions of Article 15(C) that we believe are inconsistent with South Africa's obligations and commitments under the WTO Agreement on Trade Related Aspects of Intellectual Property Rights (TRIPS).[17]

Underscoring the level of effort, the report's author, Assistant Secretary for Legislative Affairs Barbara Larkins, refers to the U.S. government's efforts as "a full court press."[18]

Although the U.S. government characterized the dispute as one that hinged on a specific interpretation of the TRIPS provisions, the struggle over intellectual property rights runs deeper than TRIPS compliance. The real struggle is over whether intellectual property rights should trump medical need in cases in which the only affordable options are not profitable for the manufacturers that own the patents.

On one hand are activists who are convinced that the overwhelming goal of policy must be the same as the rallying cry of U.S. AIDS activists in the early days of the epidemic: "Drugs into bodies." For this group, the moral answer is obvious. AIDS in the developing world, particularly sub-Saharan Africa, is a crisis of enormous proportions and like all crises deserves extraordinary measures for dealing with it. In this view, the governments of the affected countries have not only a right but a responsibility to procure medical treatments for their people by whatever means necessary. For activists, the issue is clear: The lives of people are more important than the profits of industry. Presenting the activist position to Congress in a hearing titled "U.S. Global HIV/AIDS Policy," Eric Sawyer stated:

> The administration is establishing international trade policy in a moral and intellectual vacuum—where the only thing that matters is the economic impact of trade on Western multinationals.... The Global Village is much more than a Global Market. Disowning anyone in the village—because they don't buy enough of our merchandise, because they are weak, because they don't look like us, because we are too apathetic to work for their well-being as well as our own—is not just immoral, it is a threat to public health and humanity.[19]

On the other side of the struggle is the pharmaceutical industry that develops and manufactures the medicines that are used to treat HIV itself and the opportunistic infections it causes. The industry argues that the key to innovation and research is the protection of patents and profits. According to this line of reasoning, drug development is an expensive, long-term, risky enterprise in which few products actually make it to the point of final approval. What keeps the system going and encourages companies to continue to take risks in developing new drugs is the guarantee that they will reap the rewards for the successful ones. Thus, according to this line of thought any move by countries to acquire medicines not protected by patents or sold in an unauthorized way will undermine the incentive system that is necessary for the creation of new drugs. Furthermore, according to this argument, the role of the pharmaceutical industry is best suited for what it already does: developing new drugs. It is up to government and society generally to deal with the problems of financing for these medications. The pharmaceutical manufacturers also hold out practical concerns. As administered in the United States, antiretroviral cocktails must be taken on a daily schedule and monitored closely with sophisticated tests. Failure to comply with such regimens can lead to medicine-resistant viral strains. How will developing countries provide the necessary infrastructure, the manufacturers ask, to enable people to follow these regimens and avoid the consequences of resistant viral strains?

At the same hearing at which Eric Sawyer made his statement, Dr. John Siegfried was on hand to present the position of the Pharmaceutical Research and Manufacturers of America (PhRMA), the largest U.S. pharmaceutical lobby. In the closing paragraph of his statement Siegfried quotes a prominent AIDS researcher, Dr. Thomas Coates, who had stated that introduction of the triple cocktail into regions with underdeveloped health infrastructures would be "a recipe for disaster." Thus, he concludes:

> It is neither feasible nor desirable to simply import treatment regimens from other countries into South Africa. This is true for the disease HIV/AIDS and for many other health conditions. These are complex issues that can only be addressed through collaboration involving industry, government, international organizations, patient and medical groups.[20]

Several individuals were involved in communications and meetings in Washington, D.C., and Pretoria that began even before South Africa passed Article 15(C). Ambassador Joseph, U.S. Trade Representative for Africa Rosa Whitaker, and U.S. Commerce Secretary Bill Daley all took active roles in the dispute. The most prominent U.S. government official embroiled in the dispute, however, was Vice President Al Gore. As U.S. chair of the U.S./South Africa Binational Commission (BNC), Gore was in charge of communicating directly with high-level South African government officials, including his then-counterpart, Deputy President Thabo Mbeki (who has since become president of South Africa). As the most visible figure involved on the U.S. side of the case, Gore played a prominent role in the struggle as events unfolded.

In the United States, the first phase of the struggle between the U.S. government (usually represented by the OVP) and activists who were sympathetic to the South African government position was conducted mainly through the mail. Even before South Africa passed Article 15(C), the United States had been pressuring South Africa to abandon similar policies surrounding the generic equivalent of the anti-cancer drug Taxol sold in the United States by the pharmaceutical company Bristol-Myers Squibb. On July 29, 1997, consumer advocates Ralph Nader, Robert Weissman (from the group Essential Action), and James Love (of the Consumer Project on Technology) sent the first of several letters to the vice president's office objecting to U.S. pressuring of South Africa. The letter did not achieve the hoped-for reversal of policy, nor did a second letter sent by Nader and Love on April 8, 1999.[21]

Instead, on April 30, 1999, the USTR initiated a special "out-of-cycle" review of South Africa's intellectual property policies, to be completed in September 1999. The purpose of such a review was to determine whether to implement trade sanctions against South Africa, beginning with placing South Africa on a special 301 "Watch List"—a list of countries being given heightened scrutiny by the administration to determine whether to continue with further sanctions. Vice President Gore later argued in a letter that such a move actually was a very moderate step compared to elevation of South Africa to the "Priority Foreign Government" status that the pharmaceutical companies had wanted. Such status would require resolution of the issue to the satisfaction of the United States by a certain deadline, with outright trade sanctions imposed if the deadline were not met. Many activists were infuriated by the April 30 action, and more than 300 individuals and groups involved in AIDS advocacy and public health work signed an open letter to the vice president denouncing the administration's position. At the same time, the Congressional Black Caucus entered the fray on the side of the activists and consumer organizations and wrote to Vice President Gore inquiring into the administration's actions and motives regarding South African trade policy.

In his June 25, 1999, reply to the Representative James Clayburn, chair of the Congressional Black Caucus, Gore argued that he did not have a fundamental problem with South Africa's attempts to acquire affordable medicines:

> I want you to know from the start that I support South Africa's efforts to enhance health care for its people—including efforts to engage in compulsory licensing and parallel importing of pharmaceuticals—as long as they are done in a way consistent with international agreement.[22]

This letter was greeted with mixed reactions by the AIDS and consumer activist communities. On one hand it seemed to signal a shift in the administration's position toward supporting South Africa's efforts to bring in affordable medications. On the other hand, according to the activist community the South African law already was in compliance with international agreements, but Gore's letter seemed to state at least implicitly that he was not willing to accept the law as it stood.

Although the first phase of the struggle between activists, pharmaceutical companies, and the administration was fought in a relatively subdued fashion via letters, the second phase was much more direct. It began on June 16, 1999, when Gore announced his candidacy for the Democratic nomination for the 2000 presidential election. A group of AIDS activists, many from ACT UP/Philadelphia, traveled to Carthage, Tennessee, and disrupted the kickoff of Gore's candidacy. Activists dogged his appearances at several other campaign events in Philadelphia, New York City, Washington, D.C., and even pig roasts in New Hampshire. After a summer of direct confrontations with the Democratic candidate, activists widened their range in the fall. On October 6 they held a protest against USTR Charlene Barshefsky that included a representation of her as a marionette controlled by the pharmaceutical companies. On November 17 they staged an activist takeover of her office, and on November 30—the eve of World AIDS Day—they staged a World AIDS Day Shame action targeted at President Clinton.

By the fall of 1999, activists were beginning to see some response to their efforts. Their arguments also got a boost from the spread of an antiglobalization movement that coalesced in Seattle, Washington, on November 30, 1999. Tens of thousands of protesters made their way to Seattle to voice their opposition to a world that they believed had sacrificed too many labor and human rights and environmental protections at the altar of free trade. Whereas free traders believed that a world with few or no trade barriers would create increased wealth for all countries, the protesters feared that free trade would mean that multinational corporations unfettered by national laws might impose labor and other standards of conduct on these businesses.

The case being raised by AIDS and consumer protection activists was an example of the type of scenario the protesters feared: a situation in which countries were unable to procure affordable treatments for their people because such procurements might violate the patent concerns of multinational corporations (in this case, pharmaceutical companies). Responding to the summer of intense pressure on members of his administration, the shouts of protesters in the streets, and the timing of the protests (on World AIDS Day), President Clinton backed down on South Africa. Speaking to the WTO in Seattle, he included a statement claiming that the administration would be willing to ease up on poor countries that sought to buy drugs through "parallel distributors" in other developing countries.[23] Back in Washington, D.C., the USTR and HHS Secretary Shalala offered similar announcements regarding the administration's intent to be more flexible in its approach to intellectual property and public health crises. More concretely, Barshefsky announced the removal of South Africa from the special 301 watch list.[24]

The next phase in the long saga of the official position of the U.S. government on African nations' attempts to procure essential drugs affordably occurred because of a piece of legislation before Congress. This proposed bill, the African Growth and Opportunities Act (AGOA), was very controversial in its own right. As a bill designed to lower U.S. tariffs on African goods subject to certain U.S. government conditions, it was supported by free trade advocates and denounced by those opposed to globalization. Free traders claimed that the bill would help promote economic growth in Africa while providing inexpensive goods in the United States. The antiglobalization side regarded the bill as giving the United States too much power in the U.S.-Africa relationship and thereby infringing on African sovereignty, as well as neglecting concerns over the impact of the legislation on human and labor rights. The level of controversy the bill engendered is reflected in the long time frame under which it was actively considered and the extraordinary number of changes and attempted changes that were pursued by the bill's opponents and proponents.

The AGOA was introduced in the beginning of the 106th Congress by Representative Phillip Crane, who submitted it on February 2, 1999. By the time it became Public Law 106-200 on May 18, 2000, it had been amended more than 100 times, had grown to encompass trade policy in the Caribbean Basin as well as

Africa, and had been roundly denounced by a coalition of U.S. labor unions and activists representing the sometimes overlapping agendas of debt reduction, labor and human rights, and AIDS activism. On the other side, free traders editorialized and promoted the virtues of the legislation, arguing that it gave Africa a chance to enter into a more significant economic exchange relationship with the United States.

In Congress, Representative Jesse Jackson, Jr., and Senator Russell Feingold attempted to substitute a significantly different bill for the AGOA. Their version, the Human Rights, Opportunity, Partnership and Empowerment (HOPE) Act, had several provisions that did not exist in the AGOA. The first title of the HOPE Act called for debt cancellation, and the third offered significant U.S. financial assistance, particularly for combating the AIDS epidemic. The trade provisions for Africa contained in the second title of the HOPE Act were significantly less reliant on U.S.-based conditions for granting favored status but placed considerably more emphasis on labor and human rights than the original AGOA. To the disappointment of Jackson and his backers, however, the HOPE Act never made it out of committee, and the AGOA ultimately became law.

For all of the controversy over the AGOA, however, one of the final steps of the legislation is most directly relevant to AIDS policy. Following a visit by AIDS activists, Senator Diane Feinstein, a former mayor of San Francisco, added an amendment modeled after a provision in the HOPE ACT to the AGOA. That amendment, which was cosponsored by Senator Feingold, would have formally legislated the position that AIDS advocates had been pushing for—that the United States would not interfere with actions by sub-Saharan governments to procure affordable AIDS medications as long as the governments were in compliance with TRIPS provisions.

The Feinstein amendment did not become part of the law that was ultimately passed, however, because of the stage in the legislative process known as the conference committee. When the House and Senate pass different versions of the same bill, a conference committee must create a compromise version that must be passed again by both the House and Senate. Although the conference stage obviously is a necessary part of the legislative process, it also plays a more strategic role. In conference a member of either house of Congress can quietly strip out elements or amendments to a bill that he or she opposes. In the case of AIDS legislation, conference committees have served as a "graveyard" for parts of bills that have been added by very conservative and very liberal members of Congress during the legislative process. In this case, the Feinstein-Feingold amendment became a casualty of the conference committee. The decision to strip the AGOA of the Feinstein-Feingold amendment was greeted with anger from the amendment's supporters, who accused the conferees of kowtowing to the interests of the pharmaceutical lobby behind the closed doors of the conference room. In one of several impassioned speeches on the subject, Senator Feinstein recalled her time as mayor of San Francisco during the early days of the U.S. AIDS epidemic and the lessons she learned in that role. She also made clear the level of her frustration with the conference committee and the pharmaceutical companies she believed were driving the committee. She characterized the companies as "opposed to this amendment because they want to squeeze every last drop of profit from the suffering of the millions of

HIV/AIDS victims in sub-Saharan Africa. They have shown no willingness to compromise, no willingness to enter into good faith negotiations."[25] She also threatened to use the filibuster (a Senate tactic of blocking consideration of a bill by engaging in continuous debate, thereby "talking the bill to death") to keep the Senate from voting on the version of the AGOA the conference committee had produced.

The impasse created by the struggle between the sides supporting and opposing the Feinstein-Feingold amendment was broken by a decision of President Clinton. As Clinton wrote in a letter Senator Feinstein read on the floor of the Senate, he had hoped that the issue would be decided by the inclusion of the Feinstein-Feingold amendment into the AGOA. In the wake of the conference committee's actions, however, on May 10, 2000, the president signed Executive Order 13155 containing language nearly identical to the amendment that had been stripped out of the AGOA in conference.[26]

The version of the bill created by the conference committee (without the Feinstein-Feingold amendment) had already passed the House on May 4, 2000, over the loud protest of ACT UP demonstrators who had chained themselves to their chairs in the House gallery. It passed the Senate by a vote of 77–19 on May 11, 2000, and was signed into law by the president on May 18, 2000. Free trade proponents won their law, but AIDS activists saw their goal regarding access to affordable medications formalized through Clinton's executive order.

The struggle over U.S.–African trade policy, AIDS drugs, and intellectual property rights had important spillover effects into related issues. The controversy not only raised the profile of the AIDS crisis that was occurring in the developing world, particularly sub-Saharan Africa, it also was a public relations black eye for the U.S. government and especially the international pharmaceutical industry. It also may have raised the awareness levels of government and industry themselves, motivating them to do more about the crisis as proponents for policy change provided a vivid and tragic narrative about the consequences of government and corporate positions. Motivated by some combination of self-interest and emerging awareness, the government and the pharmaceutical industry began to offer plans of their own while the AGOA debate was raging.

U.S. Government Response: Better Late than Never

The U.S. government stepped up its rhetorical and financial assistance activities significantly beginning around 1998. On World AIDS Day that year, the president directed Sandra Thurman, director of the Office of National AIDS Policy (the so-called AIDS czar), to lead a fact-finding delegation to sub-Saharan Africa and report back with recommendations. According to testimony from Thurman before Congress, this mission, conducted during the Easter recess in 1999 and accompanied by several members of Congress and their staffs, was the basis for much of the government's response.[27]

In January 2001 a widely circulated article by two Harvard researchers appearing in *The Lancet* strongly criticized the efforts of western governments, including the United States, as being greatly out of proportion with the severity of the epidemic and the giving capacity of the donor countries.[28] The article's authors, along with many activists and policy analysts, called for aid to increase by at least tenfold from its current levels. Though vastly short of this mark, U.S. financial assistance for AIDS-related activity grew significantly in 1999 and 2000. According to the Congressional Research Service, USAID reported a total of $67 million spent on fighting AIDS in Africa in fiscal year 1998 and $81 million in fiscal year 1999.

On July 19, 1999 (during the period when he was being confronted on the campaign trail by AIDS activists), Vice President Gore unveiled the administration's new AIDS plan, the Leadership in Fighting an Epidemic (LIFE) Initiative. The primary feature of the LIFE Initiative was a $100 million increase in U.S. spending on AIDS in sub-Saharan Africa and India. The money was to be divided among AIDS surveillance and prevention work (to be carried out through activities of the CDC), care for sick and orphaned children and general health care (to be directed by USAID), food assistance (carried out through existing channels but with priority for people affected by AIDS); and AIDS education in African militaries (to be carried out through the Department of Defense).[29]

The following year the administration went even further: For the first time ever it formally designated a disease as a threat to national security. Arguing that AIDS could lead to destabilization, ethnic conflicts, and outright wars, the NSC was officially directed to help craft policy solutions. The administration accompanied its statement of the threat with a call to more than double to $254 million the amount it would request from Congress to fight the pandemic overseas.

In 2001 the most substantial AIDS-related funding activity for developing countries occurred at the international level. United Nations Secretary General Kofi Annan made a public call for a new global fund. The United States, now under the leadership of a new president and party with Republican George W. Bush, pledged $200 million to the effort. Though widely touted by the administration as the first donation by a developed country, it was a very small fraction of the $2 billion that Annan had requested from the United States.

At the time of this writing, the ground is shifting rapidly around issues of AIDS in developing countries. From June 25 to 27, 2001, the United Nations convened the first special session ever held to discuss a disease. The United Nations General Assembly Special Session (UNGASS) illustrated to U.S.-based activists how far they had come in some senses and how far they had to go in others. For instance, activists were infuriated that the U.S. government selected Henry McKinnell, chief executive officer of the pharmaceutical company Pfizer and chair of PhRMA, as part of the official delegation to the meeting. During the UNGASS meeting the United States actively lobbied against discussion of health care as a right and specific mechanisms to relax patent rights to make drugs more affordable for poor countries. Some delegates, including McKinnell, even publicly argued against trying to reach the donation level the secretary general had set for the global fund. "Trying to get that much money into the system would be like pushing on a string," he said. "We couldn't spend that much money if we had it."[30] On the other hand, the idea of treatment, including antiretrovirals—which only months before been discounted as impossible to contemplate for poor countries—was openly advocated by almost all countries, including some members of the U.S. delegation.

The three major goals of AIDS foreign policy activists—debt cancellation, financial assistance, and affordable treatment—remain unrealized, although significant progress has been made. Further progress will depend, at least in part, on convincing the president, members of Congress, and more U.S. citizens that we have an obligation to extend some of what we take for granted (medicines, freedom from crushing poverty) to noncitizens in other parts of the world.

Patent Protection through Acts of Charity

Like the U.S. government, the pharmaceutical industry was thrown into a much higher level of activity by the publicity and awareness that came about because of the challenges of activists. Six giant pharmaceutical companies have featured prominently in the struggles over international AIDS policy: Boerhinger-Ingelheim, Bristol-Myers Squibb, Glaxo-Wellcome, (now GlaxoSmithKline), Hoffman-LaRoche, Merck & Co., and Pfizer. All but Pfizer manufacture one or more of the antiretroviral medications that are part of the combination therapy that is used to combat HIV directly. Pfizer makes the drug fluconazole, a medication that is used to treat several of the opportunistic infections that occur in many people with AIDS, particularly crypto-coccal meningitis (a brain infection) and thrush (which often occurs in the mouth and throat and interferes with eating).

After more than a year of being hounded by AIDS activists, *MSF*/Doctors Without Borders, and consumer groups, especially the Consumer Project on Technology, and challenged by a call from UN Secretary General Kofi Annan for new public-private partnerships to combat AIDS, the six companies began discussions via conference call in January 2000.[31] The two major issues that had to be addressed in these discussions were intellectual property rights (how to protect them) and price discounts (how much, to whom, and under what conditions). Although there was strong consensus, of course, on the need to protect intellectual property rights, the issue of price discounts was much more problematic. In fact, Pfizer is believed to have withdrawn from the six-company group because it could not accept the view that substantial price cuts were a viable company policy option.[32]

The first high-level, face-to-face meeting of the remaining five companies occurred in early March 2000. They laid out several preconditions that would have to occur before price cuts began. These preconditions included the political support of recipient countries, assumption of responsibility by international agencies for increasing the capacity of health care infrastructures, and guarantees of efficient distribution systems that would not allow diversion of drugs to other markets. They also wanted enforcement of intellectual property rights, which as a practical matter meant that they sought to eliminate the use of parallel importing and compulsory licensing. In exchange, the drug companies would be willing to acknowledge the issue of affordability for poor countries and work on solutions to that problem.

During the spring of 2000, high-level executives of the drug companies began to meet with WHO and UNAIDS, the two agencies whose support could make or break the proposal they were shaping. At the same time, industry contacts began to leak news of the plan to Michael Waldholz, a *Wall Street Journal* reporter. The UN agencies were nervous about the pharmaceutical initiative. They thought it was too vague, in terms of the preconditions it was asking for and especially in terms of what the companies would be willing to do in return. When leaders of the five companies and leaders of WHO, UNAIDS, and three other UN groups formally met for the first time, they discovered that they clearly were not on the same page. The pharmaceutical companies were eager to press forward, assuming that consensus was at hand. The agencies were deeply concerned that the price issue was still barely being mentioned, much less clearly specified. When a set of draft principles written by WHO was passed around for discussion, the pharmaceutical companies strongly objected because the issue of intellectual property protection had been left out.

Several weeks later, the concerns raised by the UN agencies still had not been addressed to their satisfaction, but a new development forced their hands. The *Wall Street Journal*, which had been sitting on the story, wanted to publish it, and on May 10 the agencies got word that the story would be broken the next day. On May 11, 2000, the *Wall Street Journal* carried a cover story by Michael Waldholz titled "Makers of AIDS Drugs Agree to Slash Prices in the Third World."[33] With no choice but to play the cards it had been dealt, UNAIDS issued a press release on the same day the story broke announcing that "a new dialogue had begun between five pharmaceutical corporations and United Nations organizations" and that "this is a promising step in a long-term process."[34]

Although the headlines in the *Wall Street Journal* and other major papers trumpeted a major breakthrough, the text of the stories revealed that details of the plan were far from determined. Only one company, Glaxo-Wellcome, had even decided on which drug it would discount and by how much. In a press release issued the same day as the breaking story and UNAIDS's press release, Glaxo-Wellcome committed itself to offering Combovir (a two-drug combination of the antiretrovirals AZT and 3TC) at approximately $2 per day (a steep reduction from the U.S. price of about $16 per day).[35]

AIDS activists and organizations that were critical of the drug companies were skeptical about the motives and the actual benefit of the announced price cuts. In its own press release issued on the same day as those of UNAIDS and Glaxo-Wellcome, *MSF*/Doctors Without Borders compared the development to "a victory, but a small one, much like an elephant giving birth to a mouse."[36] It also noted that the talks promoted only a short-term solution and recommended that a better long-term strategy would be to follow the example of Brazil, which is dealing with HIV by manufacturing its own generic drugs. Other activists wondered about the timing of the announcements. President Clinton had announced his executive order stating that the United States would no longer pressure countries not to pursue parallel importing and compulsory licensing (as long as they were TRIPS-compliant) only one day before the drug company price-cut negotiation story broke. The Thirteenth International AIDS Conference, to be held in Durban was less than two months away. Given the bad publicity the drug companies had been receiving and the preparatory work activists were doing for public demonstrations, some wondered if the announcement wasn't a sort of preemptive strike.

The premature announcement of the plan to cut prices raised expectations, but there were few details to deliver. On June 21, 2000—six weeks after the heralded announcements—UNAIDS director Piot was still pressing the companies to announce their planned discounts. All but Glaxo-Wellcome refused. In July the solidarity of the companies began to break down, with Merck leading the way in taking on its own project. It joined with the Bill Gates's philanthropic foundation to launch a $100 million program to go entirely to the tiny country (less than two million people) of Botswana. The same week, Boehringer-Ingelheim announced its own plan to provide the drug nevirapine to developing countries for the purpose of preventing HIV transmission from mother to child (recent studies had shown that nevirapine was more effective, and less costly, than AZT for this purpose).[37]

The first actual negotiation of a price cut did not occur until six months after the announcement of price cuts had been made. On October 24, 2000, the West African country of Senegal became the first African nation to successfully negotiate a deal. The deal involved two companies: Bristol-Myers Squibb and Glaxo-Wellcome. Between them, they offer drugs that can be put together to form a triple-therapy combination used in the west—Zerit and Videx from Bristol-Myers and either Crixivan or Stocrin (marketed by DuPont as Sustiva in the United States). As a result of the negotiations, the cost of triple therapy in Senegal would range from $950 to $1850 a year, as compared to a U.S. price for the same products of between $8,000 and $15,000.[38] On December 1, 2000, a deal was announced between Uganda and several pharmaceutical companies, but few specifics were given beyond the fact that several antiviral medications would be offered at negotiated discounts of as much as 66 percent and that free nevirapine would be made available to prevent mother-to-child HIV transmission.[39]

This piecemeal approach to addressing the needs of developing countries, particularly sub-Saharan Africa, was heavily criticized by activists and their allies The nevirapine announcement, for example, left many advocates angry that the company seemed to care only that babies be born HIV-negative, not that their mothers be kept alive to raise them. More generally, detractors argued that these case-by-case price breaks and giveaways constituted a deeply flawed policy approach for dealing with the problem. They felt that such programs are not sustainable; are too heavily restricted; detract from the sovereignty of the recipient nations, which must agree to conditions they may find objectionable or even unethical; and generally detract from the more desirable goal of helping countries procure for themselves an affordable and reliable supply of drugs. In October 2000, *MSF*/Doctors Without Borders released a report highlighting the foregoing problems and arguing that drug donation programs merely shift costs to taxpayers in wealthy nations. *MSF*/Doctors Without Borders argued that either differential pricing (which involves very deep discounts for developing countries to bring the price to an affordable range, as opposed to the less-drastic "discount" pricing) or simply giving developing nations the funds to procure their own generic drugs would be cheaper for taxpayers than the current policy of tax breaks for companies that donate drugs (valued at retail prices in the rich nations).[40]

In the meantime Pfizer, the company that had decided to go it alone, was having plenty of difficulties of its own. Its saga with the drug flucanazole illustrated many of the same points of contention as those for the five antiretroviral drug producers. Although Pfizer had managed to walk away from strategizing with its fellow drug companies, it was having a difficult time shaking the unwanted attention it was getting from activists in the United States and South Africa.

The push for antiretroviral medications to developing countries that the other companies offered was relatively new. Until at least 1998, the usual approach of analysts had been that precious resources had to be spent most cost-effectively, and expensive and complicated antiretroviral combination therapies did not fit that prescription. Instead, they argued, money had to be spent on prevention and testing programs. This approach softened over time as policy developers realized that, especially in areas where HIV carried enormous stigma, people had to know that getting tested would actually make them better off in some way. Few people enthusiastically line up for testing when they fear the test will result in an instruction to go home and die. Given this new insight, policymakers began to suggest a treatment approach similar to that used in the United States before antiretroviral combination therapies had been discovered—that is, treat the opportunistic infections that HIV disease facilitates, thereby prolonging life and decreasing the suffering of people with AIDS. Compared to antiretroviral combination therapies, many treatments for opportunistic infections are cheaper and simpler to administer. Pfizer's Diflucan (flucanazole) is one such treatment. Among its uses are treatment of cryptococcal meningitis and thrush.

To the activists within TAC in South Africa, therefore, flucanazole was an obvious candidate drug whose widespread use could save lives and alleviate suffering in South Africa. On March 13, 2000, TAC formally demanded that Pfizer either drastically cut its price for flucanazole in South Africa or allow South Africa to produce a generic version at an affordable price. TAC's demands were supported by the Philadelphia and Paris chapters of ACT UP, *MSF*/Doctors without Borders, and the International Gay and Lesbian Human Rights Commission, all of which issued press releases the same day supporting TAC's position. A week later, on March 21, eight members of ACT UP/New York marched into the Pfizer world headquarters to demand a meeting with chairman William J. Steere, Jr. Although they were escorted off Steere's floor by security, an account from the *New York Times* suggests that they were able to get Pfizer's attention:

> As they waited for security to drag them away, [ACT UP member] Sawyer and his comrades gleefully telephoned reporters to say where they were and why. They also notified Pfizer managers that they had scheduled a meeting to enlist the support of New York City Comptroller Alan G. Hevesi, who manages $100 billion in pension funds that hold nearly 24 million shares of Pfizer stock.[41]

Only ten days later, as TAC leaders Mark Heywood and Zackie Achmat were meeting with their lawyers in South Africa to prepare the next step against Pfizer, they were informed that Pfizer had agreed to supply free Diflucan to all people with HIV/AIDS in South Africa to treat cryptococcal meningitis. Although activists around the world savored the victory (having been given somewhat differing versions via the Internet from Achmat and the *Wall Street Journal*), Pfizer maintained that activists had not been a crucial part of its decision process:

> According to Jack Watters, Pfizer's medical director for Europe, Asia and Africa, the company had been planning just such a donation since the previous December. Asked by a reporter for documentation of that planning, he replied: "I'm not going to spend a lot of energy trying to disabuse [activists] of their notions because, frankly, I think I should put my energy into making the program work."[42]

The jubilation of activists over Pfizer's offer was short-lived, however, as details of the giveaway program began to emerge. As disappointed petitioners from Central America and Uganda quickly discovered, Pfizer was not willing to replicate its offer in other developing countries. Furthermore, on June 20, 2000, TAC of South Africa issued a press release publicizing the terms of Pfizer's offer. Not only was the offer limited to South Africa, but there were various other restrictions. These restrictions included a time-limited donation period of two-and-a-half years (coincidentally, the same time after which Pfizer's patent would expire), refusal to lower the price below R4 (U.S. $0.57) per dose for other uses, and refusal to extend the offer to treat thrush. The combined effect of the latter two conditions seemed particularly cruel to activists: Two to three times as many people suffered from thrush as meningitis, yet they would be unable to receive, or even purchase at an affordable price, the same drug that was being used to treat their fellow AIDS patients.

In response to this new information, AIDS activists again turned up the heat on Pfizer. During the summer and fall of 2000, activists staged several protests in South Africa, the United States, and France. These protests included picketing of the Pfizer factory in Pietermaritzberg, South Africa, and disruption of production at Pfizer's Touraine, France, Viagra plant by ACT UP/Paris. Members of the Boston Global Action Network staged two protests outside Pfizer's Boston research laboratories—the first with the organization Jobs With Justice on September 1 and the second in coalition with the Massachusetts Senior Action Council on October 2. Pfizer also was a primary target at the march held on the eve of the Thirteenth International AIDS Conference, and in September activists demonstrated before the UN to protest Pfizer's "bluewashing" through its inclusion in a UN "global compact" initiative. The agreement would allow the fifty companies invited to use the UN emblem in exchange for making pledges regarding their labor and environmental practices.

On World AIDS Day, December 1, 2000, Pfizer was reunited with the five antiretroviral-producing pharmaceutical companies it had sought to dissociate from when it withdrew from the March meetings over price cuts. As far as activists were concerned, the six companies had all acted in bad faith. Despite the disparity in approaches—the announced price reductions by the five antiretroviral manufacturers or the offer of a free drug in a single country by Pfizer—activists had two main criticisms. One was that neither approach represented a sustainable systematic solution to access problems. Second, and more to the point, was that as of December 1, 2000, not a single pill from any of the announced programs had actually been dispersed in any recipient country. To graphically illustrate the lack of concrete action, Health GAP used the announced theme for the day, "Men Make a Difference," as the basis of a satirical representation of the drug companies. While the group's allies at *MSF*/Doctors Without Borders released a more conventional press release arguing that the pharmaceutical companies should slash their prices in developing countries by at least 95 percent, Health GAP examined whether men do, indeed, make a difference by evaluating the six heads of the pharmaceutical companies with letter grades. Noting that in all cases, no AIDS patient had actually received a single pill of the medicine promised by the companies' plans, the resulting "report card" issued grades of "F" and "D" to the "students" that headed the six pharmaceutical giants.

Facing the Future

When George W. Bush assumed the U.S. presidency in January 2001 after eight years of the Clinton administration, one of his first actions was to place a "freeze" on the executive orders of his predecessor to determine which he might want to overturn. AIDS activists were concerned for the hard-fought specific Executive Order 13155 as well as the larger question of how many AIDS-related policies Bush might take in new directions. Many activists were particularly concerned about the level of influence that the pharmaceutical lobby might have in the new administration, and on January 26, 2001, a group within the House of Representatives sent a letter to Bush specifically asking him to preserve the Clinton executive order. To the surprise of activists, the Bush administration has agreed to leave the executive order intact.

To date, however, the new administration appears to support the pharmaceutical lobby and several of its claims. Activists were horrified at a May 2001 World Health Assembly, for instance, when HHS Secretary Tommy Thompson publicly announced to the head of the International Federation of Pharmaceutical Manufacturers, "I want you to understand I'm fighting your fight for you."[43] Similarly, Bush's head of USAID, Andrew Natsios, created deep consternation among many activists working on treatment and general advocacy for Africa with his comments that Africans could not be successfully expected to take the cocktail because they lack watches and a Western view of time.[44]

Paradoxically, although the strength of the pharmaceutical lobby may have strengthened in the transition, so too had the resolve of the opposing activist dimension. One concrete manifestation of this new resolve has been the banding together of a broad coalition of groups that collectively represented the three major policy agendas outlined at the beginning of this chapter: attention and financial aid from the U.S. government, debt reduction, and affordable drug access. On the same weekend that President Bush was being inaugurated, members of the Jubilee 2000 debt reduction movement, representatives of several African-American nongovernmental organizations, AIDS activists, and other concerned individuals and groups met for the first time in Washington, D.C. The coalition they organized, the Global AIDS Alliance (GAA), set up three complementary campaigns. The first, the $4 Billion Per Year for Africa Campaign, is dedicated to raising money from the private and public sectors to use for prevention, treatment and support of infected people, and care of AIDS orphans. The Global Right to Vital Medicines (MED4ALL) Campaign is designed to work with existing coalitions and groups to rapidly expand access to affordable AIDS medications. Finally, the Drop the Debt for AIDS campaign is assigned to work with Jubilee 2000 and other debt advocacy groups to push for rapid acceleration of debt cancellation for developing countries that are heavily affected by HIV/AIDS. In addition to the new GAA, several well-known nongovernmental organizations, most prominently Oxfam, also have launched high-profile campaigns dedicated to providing accessibility of HIV/AIDS treatments to people in developing countries, and others, including *MSF*/Doctors Without Borders and Health GAP, have renewed their commitment to treatment access campaigns.

The lives of an estimated 25 million HIV-infected people in sub-Saharan Africa are at stake, making the U.S. policy on AIDS in Africa by far the most momentous policy issue reviewed in this book. Yet the fact that it has received considerably less attention from the American government illustrates several truisms about the policy process. First, it demonstrates that the policy process is heavily influenced not by the people who are the most affected but by those who are the most organized. The relatively high level of attention this policy has gotten in recent years as opposed to the mid-1990s and earlier is a testament to the level of effort that AIDS activists have made recently. This policy area also graphically illustrates the subjective nature of policy definition. At any given time, many items on the government agenda are competing for attention. Those that get that attention do so not because of any numerical measure of absolute importance but on the basis of how strategically policy players have presented their issues.

How the struggle that has taken shape between corporate interests and grassroots advocates will be resolved remains to be seen. Similarly, it is impossible to predict with certainty how and to what extent the new presidential administration and Congress will engage in the struggle. One thing we can say with certainty is that the original problems on which the struggle is based are growing steadily worse. As more and more people grow sick and die, the level of human suffering caused by AIDS in sub-Saharan Africa and other developing regions and the inability of these countries' governments to cope financially, logistically, and medically with the crisis will only increase. Although there have been important policy shifts relative to the United States' policy role in previous decades, a far more drastic response is needed if this country is to play a meaningful and helpful role in the future of sub-Saharan Africa.

CHAPTER 7

Conclusion: Struggling toward the Future

On January 28, 2001, the *New York Times Magazine* carried an extensive story with an impossibly long subtitle.[1] That subtitle—"Patent Laws Are Malleable. Patients Are Educable. Drug Companies Are Vincible. The World's AIDS Crisis Is Solvable"—was a preamble to the headline: "Look at Brazil." It also was obviously a political argument. In the story, writer Tina Rosenberg outlined the drug treatment system of Brazil, which since 1997 has been committed to the goal of providing, free of charge, triple cocktails to any Brazilian who needs them. (Recall that in the United States, the richest country in the world, there are waiting lists in some states for ADAP coverage for the same triple cocktail.) The Brazilian system achieves the same levels of compliance to the strict medical regimen as in the United States, despite the fact that Brazil is a poor country that was starting with a poor health care infrastructure and despite the fact that only very recently have people in the rest of the world even begun to acknowledge the possibility of providing antiretroviral drugs in poor countries.

Rosenberg cites three keys to Brazil's successes. The first, political commitment to spend the money needed to run the treatment program nationwide, has been true even in the face of severe budget constraints in early 1999. The second, an aggressive AIDS prevention program, has included provision of millions of free condoms to activists groups for distribution. Prevention has been complemented by the third crucial element: Brazil's formulation of its patent laws to allow for the manufacture of generic equivalents of brand-name elements of the AIDS cocktail.[2] In the Brazilian system people have an incentive to get tested because treatment is free and treatment lowers viral loads, making people less infectious to others.

Rosenberg's appraisal of Brazil's program—that it offers a viable solution to the raging AIDS pandemic among poor people, as an example of what one country has done and as a possible source of cheap medication—is profoundly at odds with the U.S. government's position as well as the wishes of the world's large pharmaceutical companies. The U.S. response to Brazil's innovations was to file a complaint against Brazil with the WTO. Although that case was dropped during the UN Special Session on AIDS in June 2001, the United States has maintained its opposition to the Brazilian approach of providing generically produced antiretroviral drugs to poor people in poor countries.

Brazil's policies raise profound questions for the direction of U.S. foreign and domestic policy. Brazil has maintained a commitment to AIDS care and prevention that has been highly responsive to the country's gay community and poor population. In the United States, the gay community organized itself into activist groups and service organizations and became a force to be reckoned with. As AIDS in the United States increasingly becomes a disease of poor people and minority groups, however, whether the government and society in general will continue to give AIDS high priority remains to be seen.

To AIDS activists, there are reasons for concern. The federal government's long-standing refusal to support needle-exchange programs (even during the more liberal Clinton administration); the continuous struggles during the Ryan White CARE Act authorizations over whether to give money to the most well-established or the most needy demographic groups; and the gap between the need for and the supply of antiretroviral medications for poor people through ADAPs are examples of policy decisions that suggest commitment levels to poor people and racial minorities are not strong. Furthermore, the rules of politics as exemplified in the pages of this book suggest that it will be very hard for poor people, who are neither tightly organized nor well-resourced, to achieve their policy aims against opponents who have the upper hand organizationally and financially.

In terms of international policy, the challenge Brazil raises for the United States is even more direct. The demographics of the epidemic are inexorably moving in a single direction: As more time that passes, AIDS increasingly becomes a disease of poor and dispossessed people. This observation is true within rich nations such as the United States, where AIDS and the challenges of dealing with it are increasingly located in poor minority communities. It is even truer around the world: AIDS's greatest growth is in the poorest nations and regions. The U.S. government will increasingly be forced to take sides between commercial interests that are dedicated to maintaining systems of protection of property, especially intellectual property, and humanitarian interests that are concerned with saving lives.

Lessons from the AIDS Policy Realm

The realm of AIDS policy, like most policy areas, is always changing because the features of the epidemic and the policy players are in a constant state of flux. Policy formulation began when no one had any idea what HIV was, let alone what to do for someone infected by it. Since then, remarkable (but expensive) strides have been made. We can now detect the presence of HIV in blood and a host of other body fluids. We know how HIV is transmitted, as well as how it is not. We can treat the opportunistic infections that occur with a compromised immune system and, provided resistance doesn't develop, keep the immune system from becoming compromised by prescribing combination therapy. We can address the social and support needs of people through programs such as the Ryan White CARE Act. Yet none of this progress has reduced the controversy. If anything, it has created more.

Chapters 2 through 6 cover issues people who are affected by AIDS consider to be very important. They also illustrate policy dynamics that go beyond the specifics of AIDS policy, however. Each of the policy chapters in this book is designed to illustrate a larger policy dilemma that applies to many other policies outside the realm of AIDS. Chapter 2 is about *policy definition* (in this case, as a right or a market commodity). Chapter 3 looks at the perennial policy challenges inherent in the task of *regulation*. Chapter 4 examines the problem of *competing values* in policy selection. Chapter 5 illustrates the problems of *distributive politics,* and chapter 6 looks at the difficult policy dilemma of *membership* in policy distribution.

The substance of chapter 2—medical treatment for people with AIDS— traces a story of medical advances, personal self-empowerment, and rising health care costs. It also is about a much more fundamental issue, however. The opposing sides in this particular struggle have difficulty finding common ground because they have a fundamental disagreement over the nature of medical care. Proponents of greater access and affordability of medical treatment options press for those goals in part because they believe that such access should be available to all as a matter of course. Health care, from this point of view, is a right. The other side argues that the demands for treatment must be balanced with sensitivity toward companies manufacturing the products being demanded. They do so because they regard health care as a market good that is bought and sold like any other. This struggle over the nature of health care—as right or commodity—is mirrored in many other policy debates. If health care is a right the government has an obligation to provide it, or at least make sure it is available and affordable to everyone. If it is a commodity, the government need only make certain that the rules in the marketplace between buyers and sellers are reasonably fair. The policy debate over what constitutes a right and what is merely a market commodity has been an enduring source of division in American government and society.

Chapter 6 asks the question (is health care a right or a commodity?) again, but with a twist. Do the same rules apply beyond a country's borders? If people in the United States should be able to expect government assistance to provide them with life-saving drugs, should noncitizens have the same expectations? Should the rules that operate within a country (for consumers and producers of medical products) extend beyond its borders? If not, should people outside the United States be able to expect at least a minimum level of financial support and resources, particularly medicines, by virtue of our common humanity? Thus, chapter 6 is about the concept of membership. That is, how far should benefits extend—to citizens of a single country or to all members of a global community? Again, this question is a knotty problem not merely for AIDS activists but for human rights advocates, environmentalists, and all sorts of other groups seeking to explore the issue of whether citizenship or common humanity should be the criterion we should use for deciding the expectations people should have of governments.

Although chapter 3 specifically addresses HIV contamination of the U.S. blood supply, more generally it explores the challenges of regulation. Regulation is always about government's application of rules to an industry to make its products or production methods in some way more advantageous to consumers— cheaper, cleaner, or, in the case of the blood supply, safer. Because such regulation necessarily imposes costs on the industry, the industry can be expected to resist attempts to impose it. Whether the government and consumers react with strength or weakness is a perennial question in regulatory politics; as with the blood supply, strong regulation often does not come about until after serious damage has occurred.

Balancing the competing needs of consumers and industry is a matter of setting boundaries and limits, as well as assigning levels of responsibility. All of these activities will dissatisfy at least one side in the struggle: the one that is asked to bear more costs or to take more responsibility. Thus, regulatory politics guarantee a continuous struggle between consumers and producers to try to get the government to shift the cost and responsibility to the other side.

The central issue in chapter 4 is not material costs but the strength of competing values. Although money and financial considerations are important determinants of our individual actions and collective policy choices, chapter 4 demonstrates that policy is not only about money. Sometimes the most hard-fought struggles are waged not about our pocketbooks but about our values. Almost none of the people who have fought over condom distribution in the schools, needle exchanges, newborn HIV testing, or other prevention strategies entered the fray because of monetary motivations. They chose to fight because they felt that privacy, family values, societal norms, or some other deeply felt values were in danger and had to be protected. There are many other such value-driven debates going on in the United States. Abortion, censorship, the death penalty, gun control: These controversies are not primarily policy struggles over money. They are struggles over deeply held values, and they will continue as long as there are deeply committed proponents on both sides of these questions.

Whereas chapter 4 makes the important point that not all policy battles are waged over the bottom line, chapter 5 concedes that some are. Chapter 5 is centrally concerned with distributive politics: the tough challenge of assigning resources to competing groups. In chapter 5 we are reminded of a few truisms about the way in which distributive politics operate. One is that distributions reflect the strength and organizational levels of the groups that exist when the distribution is originally made. In the case of the Ryan White CARE Act, strong community-based organizations and well-organized cities got more resources in the initial distribution established by the new law. The same dynamic occurs in other distributions, however, whether they involve military spending, entitlement programs, or decisions about where to put roads and sidewalks.

The other truism that is amply illustrated by the Ryan White CARE Act is that it is easier to create a distributive program than it is to alter the distribution once it has been made. To an outsider it may seem irrational that spending on AIDS has not followed the geographic and demographic trends of the disease more closely. The careful observer sees, however, that once a distribution has begun, groups that benefit have an interest in not altering the distribution. This observation is true for policy areas far beyond AIDS, such as farm subsidies, weapons acquisitions, and government grants.

The Big Picture

In chapter 1 I argue against a model of government policymaking that suggests that government examines a group of options, finds the best choice by some objective standard, and implements it. Such a model assumes a high level of rationality and a small number of policy decision makers. It also leaves out at least three elements that AIDS policy illustrates are tremendously important. To have a more complete picture of policymaking, whether the policy in question concerns AIDS or any of dozens of other subjects, we must look at the three distinct aspects of policymaking I introduce at the very beginning of the book:

1. **The role of organization.** The story of policy struggle is the story of organization. Some of the most compelling stories from the realm of AIDS policymaking are interesting because they are modern-day David-and-Goliath tales. The tiny hemophilia community successfully sought retribution from the U.S. government and the fractionators, and small groups of AIDS activists have successfully pressed claims against powerful multinational pharmaceutical corporations. The key to these successes was not luck (though perhaps that helped). It was organization. In the policy process, organized groups have power. Moreover, although money certainly is a useful commodity, it is not the only currency in the work of organization. A shared vision, strong ties within a group, deeply held values—all of these have been valuable tools that have been used by groups such as the hemophilia community and ACT UP to accomplish goals against a competing side with greater monetary resources.

2. **The role of values.** Objectively speaking, there have been major advances in our technological abilities to deal with HIV and AIDS. We now have medicines that have turned AIDS from an inevitably fatal diagnosis to a chronic condition. We know a great deal about how it is spread and how to prevent that spread. We have a great deal of cumulative information about the most common problems faced by people infected with HIV. Yet many of the fundamental controversies around AIDS that emerged even before the disease had a name—how to conduct prevention efforts, how generous to be with treatment options, how much decision and policymaking power to give to infected people—still rage on. This continuing controversy reflects the fact that technological solutions cannot solve political problems. Technological advances give us more tools and skills for problem solving, but they cannot by themselves change the values we apply to problems. Most of the values that were in place at the beginning of the epidemic— such as concerns over privacy for some people, concerns for family values for others—remain in place. The same dynamic obtains in policy areas beyond AIDS. Our world changes more rapidly than our values do. Our values drive the positions we take, whether the issue is AIDS, military spending, school prayer, or any other of the dozens of policy areas that affect our lives every day.

3. **The problem of inflicting costs and changing distributions.** It would be foolish to argue that policy is only about values. The central task of politics is distribution—dividing the costs and benefits of policies among the many groups seeking to gain the benefits and avoid the costs. It is important to remember, however, that in this area of activity, not all types of distribution are created equal. Battles over regulation of the blood supply, changing the rules of international trade regarding AIDS medicines, and redistributing money for the Ryan White CARE Act all point to one simple truism: It is much easier to establish policies that provide benefits (whether in the form of favorable rules or outright

financial gains) than it is to restructure those policies. Given the equally simple reality that situations change (for example, when demographics shift or new problems surface), we should be able to predict that redistribution, with all its attendant problems, will always be a challenge for the policy process.

The dynamics of HIV/AIDS policymaking are not unique, though they are dramatic. The same underlying pressures that create policy struggles have been at work in these issues. These policy struggles have been unusual in their visibility, however. The struggles have made for good press: Demonstrations, confrontations in the streets, and new ways of framing old issues all attract media attention. As the AIDS pandemic moves increasingly into the global arena, these policy dynamics will play out again, but the problems will be even more important, with many more lives and cultural values at stake. As this book seeks to illustrate, policy is not handed down from detached governments and administrators. It is created through the struggles of determined and organized individuals motivated by deeply held values. The future direction of the AIDS pandemic, as well as the future direction of other pressing policy problems, will be determined by the groups that join the struggle and the values for which they choose to fight.

Notes

Chapter 1

1. For an excellent outline of this policy approach as well as an alternative view, see Deborah Stone, *Policy Paradox: The Art of Political Decision Making* (New York: W.W. Norton, 1997).

2. Probably the most widely credited articulation of this view is David Truman, *The Governmental Process* (New York: Knopf, 1951).

3. This problem was first suggested by Mancur Olson, *The Logic of Collective Action* (Cambridge, Mass.: Harvard University Press, 1965).

4. Robert Putnam, *Bowling Alone: The Collapse and Revival of American Community* (New York: Simon & Schuster, 2000).

5. See Allan Brandt, *No Magic Bullet: A Social History of Venereal Disease in the United States Since 1880* (New York: Oxford University Press, 1985), for a discussion of these dynamics with respect to sexually transmitted diseases.

6. Here we should note a technical distinction. In this book I refer to the AIDS *epidemic* and the AIDS *pandemic*. An epidemic occurs when the incidence of a disease exceeds the expected rate within a given area. A pandemic is a multinational epidemic. Thus, when I discuss the problems of AIDS within the United States, I refer to the AIDS epidemic; when I talk about AIDS worldwide, I refer to it as a pandemic.

7. For a more detailed description of these events, see Patricia Siplon, "Action Equals Life: The Power of Community in AIDS Political Activism" (Ph.D. diss., Brandeis University, 1997).

8. Before we are too quick to make assumptions that people who use drugs are inherently unable to organize, however, we might look to other countries such as the Netherlands, where drug addicts formed groups that conducted needle distribution to help slow the spread of hepatitis before AIDS had even made its appearance.

9. For an excellent explanation of the complicated relationship between the African-American community and AIDS politics and policies, see Cathy J. Cohen, *The Boundaries of Blackness* (Chicago: University of Chicago Press, 1997).

10. Centers for Disease Control, "Pneumocystic Pneumonia—Los Angeles," *Morbidity and Mortality Weekly Report* 30, no. 21 (5 June 1981): 250–52.

11. A discussion of the CDC's deliberations on how to present the report can be found in Randy Shilts, *And the Band Played On: Politics, People and the AIDS Epidemic* (New York: St. Martin's Press, 1987), 68–69.

12. Gerald M. Oppeheimer, "Causes, Cases and Cohorts: The Role of Epidemiology in the Historical Construction of AIDS," in *AIDS: The Making of a Chronic Disease*, ed. Elizabeth Fee and Daniel Fox (Berkeley: University of California Press, 1992), 53.

13. Ibid., 59.

14. Don Des Jerlais, Samuel Friedman, and Jo Sotheran, "The First City: HIV Among Intravenous Drug Users in New York City," in Fee and Fox, *AIDS: The Making of a Chronic Disease*, 283.

15. Gerald Oppenheimer, "In the Eye of the Storm: The Epidemiological Construction of AIDS," in *AIDS: The Burdens of History*, ed. Elizabeth Fee and Daniel Fox (Berkeley: University of California Press, 1988), 273–77.

16. Steven Epstein, *Impure Science: AIDS, Activism and the Politics of Knowledge* (Berkeley: University of California Press, 1996), 55.

17. My account of Gallo's relationship to the discovery of HIV is taken from Epstein, *Impure Science*, 67–74.

18. Shilts, *And the Band Played On*, 450–51.

19. Epstein, *Impure Science*, 71; Shilts, *And the Band Played On*, 528–29.

20. Epstein, *Impure Science*, 131–35.

21. Peter H. Duesberg and Bryan J. Ellison, "Is the AIDS Virus a Science Fiction? Immunosuppressive Behavior, Not HIV, May Be the Cause of AIDS," *Policy Review* (summer 1990): 40–51.

22. Marlene Cimons, "Rethinking Priorities on AIDS: The Infections that Prey on Those with Damaged Immune Systems Have Been Targets of Little Interest to Researchers. The Emphasis Has Been Finding a Cure for the Syndrome," *Los Angeles Times*, 9 April 1990, A1.

Chapter 2

1. A lively description of these and many other demonstrations appears in Douglas Crimp and Adam Rolston, *AIDS Demo Graphics* (Seattle: Bay Press, 1990), 26–29.

2. An account of this story, told primarily from activist Michael Callen's perspective, appears in Bruce Nussbaum, *Good Intentions* (New York: Penguin Books, 1990), 107–10.

3. Ibid., 34–35.

4. This process is described in Peter S. Arno and Karen L. Feiden, *Against the Odds: The Story of AIDS, Drug Development, Politics and Profit* (New York: Harper Collins, 1992), 261–65. A perspective from former FDA director David Kessler—who ultimately was responsible for the results—is given in David A. Kessler, "The Regulation of Investigational Drugs," *New England Journal of Medicine* 320, no. 5 (2 February 1989): 281–88. The FDA has described the process as well and has posted it at www.fda.gov.cder/handbook/develop.htm.

5. Nussbaum, *Good Intentions*, 38–39.

6. Arno and Feiden, *Against the Odds*, 40; Nussbaum, *Good Intentions*, 40–41.

7. Nussbaum, *Good Intentions*, 43–44.

8. Robert Yarchoan et al., "Administration of 3'–Azido-3'–Deoxythymidine, an Inhibitor of HTLV-III/LAV Replication, to Patients with AIDS or AIDS-Related Complex," *Lancet* 1, no. 8481 (15 March 1986): 575–80.

9. The first published results of the Phase II trials appear as two articles published in the *New England Journal of Medicine*. See Margaret Fischl et al., "The Efficacy of Azidothymidine (AZT) in the Treatment of Patients with AIDS and AIDS-Related Complex," and Douglas Richmond et al., "The Toxicity of Azidothymidine (AZT) in the Treatment of Patients with AIDS and AIDS-Related Complex," *New England Journal of Medicine* 317, no. 4 (23 July 1987): 185–97.

10. Arno and Feiden, *Against the Odds*, 43.

11. John Lauritzen, *Poison by Prescription: The AZT Story* (New York: Asklepios, 1990), 30. Similar weaknesses are pointed out by Steven Epstein, *Impure Science: AIDS, Activism, and the Politics of Knowledge* (Berkeley: University of California Press, 1996), 202–03.

12. Fischl et al., "Efficacy of Azidothymidine," 186.

13. This information and the discussion between members of Congress and Burroughs Wellcome about pricing appear in the transcript of the Subcommittee on Health and Environment of House Committee on Energy and Commerce, *AIDS Issues (Part I): Cost and Availability of AZT*, 100th Cong., 1st sess., 10 March 1987, 8.

14. Ibid., 26.

15. Gina Kolata, "Strong Evidence Discovered that AZT Holds Off AIDS," *New York Times*, 4 August 1989, A1.

16. Philip Hilts, "AIDS Drug's Maker Cuts Price by 20%, Cites Mounting Demands and Protests by Advocates," *New York Times*, 19 September 1989, A1.

17. Financial Desk, "Drug Maker Rejects Pleas," *New York Times*, 6 September 1989, D18.

18. Editorial, "AZT's Inhuman Cost," *New York Times*, 28 August 1989, A16.

19. Crimp and Rolston, *AIDS Demo Graphics*, 117.

20. Hilts, "AIDS Drug's Maker Cuts Price by 20%."

21. Epstein, *Impure Science*, 299–300.

22. Jean-Pierre Aboulker and Ann Marie Swart, "Preliminary Analysis of the Concorde Trial, *Lancet* 341 (3 April 1993): 889–90.

23. Gina Kolata, "Federal Delay in Lowering Standard for Doses of AIDS Drug Is Assailed," *New York Times*, 27 December 1989, A1.

24. Gifford Leoung et al., "Aerolized Pentamidine for Prophylaxis Against *Pneumocystis Carinii* Pneumonia: The San Francisco Community Prophylaxis Trial," *New England Journal of Medicine* 323, no. 12 (20 September 1990): 769.

25. Arno and Feiden, *Against the Odds*, 85.

26. Letter from National Organization for Rare Disorders to Lymphomed, submitted for the record by Brain Tambim, speaking before Subcommittee of House Committee on Government Operations, *Therapeutic Drugs for AIDS: Development, Testing and Availability*, 100th Cong., 2nd sess., 28 April 1988, 436.

27. Ibid., 441.

28. Arno and Feiden, *Against the Odds*, 89.

29. Beverly Merz, "Aerolized Pentamidine Promising in Pneumcystis Therapy, Prophylaxis," *Journal of the American Medical Association* 259, no. 22 (10 June 1988): 3223–24.

30. Arno and Feiden, *Against the Odds*, 94.

31. A complete account of the trial is given in Leoung, "Aerolized Pentamidine for Prophylaxis," 769–75.

32. Arno and Feiden, *Against the Odds*, 112–13.

33. Subcommittee of House Committee on Government Operations, *Therapeutic Drugs for AIDS*.

34. Merz, "Aerolized Pentamidine Promising in Pneumcystis Therapy, Prophylaxis," 3224.

35. Arno and Feiden, *Against the Odds*, 65–66.

36. Gina Kolata, "Company Devised AIDS Drug Test Partly as Sales Tool," *New York Times*, 10 January 1991, B9.

37. Arno and Feiden, *Against the Odds*, 118.

38. Gena Corea, *The Hidden Malpractice: How American Medicine Mistreats Women as Patients and Professionals* (New York: Harper and Row, 1985).

39. Ibid., 299–302.

40. For examples of documentation of the inspiration that women activists, particularly lesbians, provided to the self-empowerment end of AIDS activism, see Nancy E. Stoller, "Lesbian Involvement in the AIDS Epidemic: Changing Roles and Generational Differences," in *Women Resisting AIDS: Feminist Strategies of Empowerment*, ed. Beth E. Schneider and Nancy E. Stoller (Philadelphia: Temple University Press, 1995), 270–85, and Maxine Wolf, "AIDS and Politics: Transformation of Our Movement," in ACT UP/NY Women and AIDS Book Group, *Women, AIDS and Activism* (Boston: South End Press, 1990), 233–37.

41. Given the importance of these principles for the self-empowerment movement, it is not surprising that they are still widely available. See Advisory Committee of the People With AIDS, "The Denver Principles," 1983, reprinted in *Women, AIDS and Activism,* 239–40, and available online at www.actupny.org/documents/Denver.html and www.beingalivela.org/news598/598_denvp.html (last accessed September 20, 2001).

42. Ibid.

43. Renee Sabatier, *Blaming Others: Prejudice, Race and Worldwide AIDS* (Santa Cruz, Calif.: New Society Publishers, 1988), 144.

44. Nussbaum, *Good Intentions,* 110.

45. Gerald J. Stine, *AIDS Update 2000* (Upper Saddle River, N.J.: Prentice Hall, 2000), 83.

46. David Brown, "U.S. Advocates Triple Therapy to Fight AIDS: Agency Guidelines Urge Aggressive Treatment," *Washington Post,* 20 June 1997, A1.

47. The living document has been just that. It was modified in January 2000 and on February 5, 2001. Current and archived versions are made available through the HIV/AIDS Treatment Information Service and can be accessed online at http://hivatis.org/trtgdlns.html (last accessed February 14, 2001).

48. Centers for Disease Control, "Table 21. AIDS Cases and Deaths, by Year and Age Group, through December 2000, United States," *HIV/AIDS Surveillance Report* 12, no. 4 (24 September 2001). Available online at www.cdc.gov/hiv/stats/hasr1202/table21.htm (last accessed 27 December 2001).

49. As I discuss in chapter 6, this is the price in the United States. It is possible to produce the same combination and sell it for a very small fraction of this price (under $500), but doing so requires licensing of generic manufacturers, and current trade law works strongly against this possibility.

50. General Accounting Office, *HIV/AIDS Drugs: Funding Implications of New Combination Therapies for Federal and State Programs* (GAO/HHS-99-2), 14 October 1998, Letter Report.

51. Dan Levy, "Millions Fail to Get Vital AIDS Medicines; UCSF Finds Medicaid Isn't Delivering in 4 Big States," *San Francisco Chronicle,* 4 November 2000, A1. The original Associated Press story was circulated as Laura Meckler, "Some AIDS Patients Get the Wrong Drugs," 3 November 2000.

52. Levy, "Millions Fail to Get Vital AIDS Medicines."

53. These arguments are summarized in Bruce D. Walker and Nesli Basgoz, "Treat HIV Like Other Infections—Treat It," *Journal of the American Medical Association* 280, no. 1 (1 July 1998): 91–93.

54. William J. Burman, Randall R. Reeves, and David L. Cohn, "The Case for Conservative Management of Early HIV Disease," *Journal of the American Medical Association* 280, no. 1 (1 July 1998): 93–95.

55. Jeff Getty, "Drug Holiday Forum Gets Record Crowd," *Bay Area Reporter,* 5 May 2000.

Chapter 3

1. Michael Davon, letter to Senator James Jeffords, 10 September 1998; www.web-depot.com/mailing-lists/archives (last accessed 10 September 1998).

2. For a vivid account of this international system of plasma collection and processing, see Douglas Starr, *Blood: An Epic History of Medicine and Commerce* (New York: Alfred A. Knopf, 1998), 231–41.

3. Institute of Medicine, *HIV and the Blood Supply: An Analysis of Crisis Decisionmaking* (Washington, D.C.: National Academy Press, 1995), 37.

4. Susan Resnick, *Blood Saga: Hemophilia, AIDS and the Survival of a Community*, (Berkeley: University of California Press, 1999), 79–83.

5. Ibid., 96.

6. Ibid., 97.

7. Institute of Medicine, *HIV and the Blood Supply*, 44–45.

8. Public Health Service Committee on Opportunistic Infections in Patients with Hemophilia, "Summary Report on Open Meeting of PHS Committee on Opportunistic Infections in Patients with Hemophilia" (U.S. Public Health Service, Washington, D.C., 1982, photocopy).

9. National Hemophilia Foundation, *Hemophilia Newsnotes*, 14 July 1982.

10. National Hemophilia Foundation, "Medical Bulletin #10/ Chapter Advisory #13," *Hemophilia Information Exchange: AIDS Update*, 24 January 1984.

11. National Hemophilia Foundation, "Chapter Advisory #14," *Hemophilia Information Exchange: AIDS Update*, 3 February 1984, 1.

12. National Hemophilia Foundation, "Medical Bulletin #11," *Hemophilia Information Exchange: AIDS Update*, 30 January 1984.

13. Starr, *Blood*, 271.

14. Ibid.

15. Ibid., 273.

16. American Association of Blood Banks, American Red Cross, and Council of Community Blood Centers, "Joint Statement of Acquired Immune Deficiency Syndrome (AIDS) Related to Transfusion," 13 January 1983 (photocopy), 2.

17. Starr, *Blood*, 275.

18. Memorandum from Dr. Cumming to Mr. DeBeaufort, 5 February 1983, American Red Cross National Headquarters, 3.

19. Memorandum from S. J. Ojala re: "National Hemophilia Foundation/Industry Strategy Meeting on AIDS, January 14, 1983, New York City," Cutter Laboratories, 17 January 1983.

20. National Center for Drugs and Biologics, "Recommendations to Decrease the Risk of Transmitting Acquired Immune Deficiency Syndrome (AIDS) from Blood Donors," 24 March 1983 (Food and Drug Administration, Bethesda, Md.) and National Center for Drugs and Biologics, "Source Material Used to Manufacture Certain Plasma Derivatives," 24 March 1983 (Food and Drug Administration, Bethesda, Md.).

21. Starr, *Blood*, 292.

22. Institute of Medicine, *HIV and the Blood Supply*, 75.

23. Starr, *Blood*, 295.

24. Ibid., 297.

25. Ronald Bayer, "Blood and AIDS in America: The Making of a Catastrophe," in *Blood Feuds: AIDS, Blood and the Politics of Medical Disaster*, ed. Erik Feldman and Ronald Bayer (New York: Oxford University Press, 1999), 30–31.

26. Institute of Medicine, *HIV and the Blood Supply*, 158.

27. Bayer, "Blood and AIDS in America," 30.

28. Institute of Medicine, *HIV and the Blood Supply*, 151.

29. Ibid., 148.

30. Biological Coordinating Committee, "Confidential Memorandum," Cutter Laboratories, 20 March 1986.

31. Starr, *Blood,* 297.

32. Ibid.

33. Institute of Medicine, *HIV and the Blood Supply,* 156.

34. Ibid., 158.

35. Bayer, "Blood and AIDS in America," 32.

36. Ibid., 33.

37. Institute of Medicine, *HIV and the Blood Supply,* 21.

38. This number includes four categories from the CDC Surveillance Report: adult/ adolescent hemophilia/coagulation disorder (4,911); adult/adolescent sex with person with hemophilia (429); pediatric hemophilia/coagulation disorder (234); and [child of] mother with/at risk for HIV infection through sex with person with hemophilia (29). All numbers are taken from Centers for Disease Control and Prevention, *HIV/AIDS Surveillance Report* 10, no. 2 (1998), 14.

39. Ibid.

40. Timothy Cook and David Colby, "The Mass Mediated Epidemic," in *AIDS: The Making of a Chronic Disease,* ed. Elizabeth Fee and Daniel Fox (Berkeley: University of California Press, 1992), 84–122.

41. Greg Haas, "Denial, Anger, Destruction and Unity," *Common Factor* 7 (February 1994): 20.

42. Resnick, *Blood Saga,* 195.

43. Corey Dubin, interview with author, 28 July 1999.

44. Ibid.

45. Jan Hamilton, "The Hemophilia Federation: A New National Organization," *Common Factor* 5 (June 1993): 1.

46. Ibid.

47. Greg Haas, "Time for People with Hemophilia and HIV to Act Up?" *Common Factor* 4 (April 1993): 18.

48. Bayer, "Blood and AIDS in America," 41.

49. Institute of Medicine, *HIV and the Blood Supply,* vi.

50. Ibid., 194.

51. Ibid., 194–95.

52. Ibid., 95.

53. Ibid., 229–30.

54. Ibid., 6.

55. Bayer, "Blood and AIDS in America," 39.

56. Resnick, *Blood Saga,* 176.

57. Bayer, "Blood and AIDS in America," 47.

58. Starr, *Blood,* 342.

59. Jonathan Wadleigh, "NHF Opposes Class Certification," *Common Factor* 8 (June 1994), 1.

60. *In the Matter of Rhone-Poulenc Rorer, Inc.,* 51 F. 3d 1293 (7th Cir. 1995), 1297.

61. Barry Meier, "Blood, Money and AIDS: Hemophiliacs Are Split; Liability Cases Bogged Down in Disputes" *New York Times,* 11 June 1996, D1.

62. Bayer, "Blood and AIDS in America," 52.

63. Dana Kuhn, e-mail correspondence to hemophilia listserve (hemophilipa-support@web-depot.com), 22 October 2000.

64. House Judiciary Committee, *Report to Accompany H.R. 1023*, 105th Cong., 2d sess., 1998, 7.

65. Dave Cavanaugh, "COTT Washington Update," posted to hemophilia listserve (hemophilipa-support@web-depot.com), 15 December 2000.

66. Sean Donohue (legislative aide to Senator James Jeffords), telephone conversation with author, 16 January 2001.

67. G. Pascal Zachary, "Users Want Say in Oversight of Blood," *Wall Street Journal*, 10 June 1994, B1.

Chapter 4

1. *Congressional Record*, 100th Cong., 1st sess., 14 October 1987, 27753.

2. Ibid., 27754.

3. Ibid., 27757.

4. Ibid., 27760.

5. Gerald J. Stein, *AIDS Update 2000* (Upper Saddle River, N.J.: Prentice Hall, 2000), 217.

6. C. Everett Koop, *Koop: The Memoirs of America's Family Doctor* (New York: Random House, 1991), 226.

7. Ibid.

8. From "Understanding AIDS: A Message from the Surgeon General," Appendix A in Koop, *Memoirs of a Family Doctor*.

9. Pieces of Kramer's earliest messages are quoted in Ronald Bayer, *Private Acts, Social Consequences: AIDS and the Politics of Public Health* (New Brunswick, N.J.: Rutgers University Press, 1989), 23. See also Randy Shilts, *And the Band Played On: Politics, People and the AIDS Epidemic* (New York: St. Martins Press, 1987), 108–09.

10. Bayer, *Private Acts, Social Consequences*, 24.

11. Perhaps the most famous statement in this debate was the essay by Callen and Richard Berkowitz, "We Know Who We Are," published in the *New York Native* in December 1982. This essay drew a clear line connecting promiscuity and AIDS, and argued for much more decisive behavioral changes. See Shilts, *And the Band Played On*, 209–10.

12. Shilts, *And the Band Played On*, 167.

13. A discussion of these findings appears in Gerald M. Oppenheimer, "Causes, Cases, and Cohorts: The Role of Epidemiology in the Historical Construction of AIDS," in *AIDS: The Making of a Chronic Disease*, ed. Elizabeth Fee and Daniel Fox (Berkeley: University of California Press, 1992), 49–83.

14. Bayer, *Private Acts, Social Consequences*, 211.

15. Ibid.

16. Ibid., 212.

17. These estimates from the Institute of Medicine, *The Hidden Epidemic* (Washington, D.C.: National Academy Press, 1997), and Alan Guttmacher Institute, *Sex and America's Teenagers* (New York and Washington, D.C.: Alan Guttmacher Institute, 1994), respectively, are quoted in Centers for Disease Control, "Trends in Sexual Risk Behaviors Among High School Students—United States, 1991–1997," *Mortality and Morbidity Weekly Report* 47, no. 36 (18 September 1998): 749–52; available at www.cdc.gov/nchstp/dstd/MMWRs/Trends_Risk_Behaviors_HS_students.htm (last accessed 8 October 2000).

18. American Social Health Association, "Teenagers Know More Than Adults About STDs, but Knowledge Among Both Groups Is Low," *STD News* 3 (winter 1996): 1, 5.

19. Henry J. Kaiser Family Foundation, "Sex Education in the U.S.: Policy and Politics," *Issue Update*, September 2000, 1. Available at www.kff.org (last accessed 8 October 2000).

20. Kaiser Family Foundation, "Sex Education in the U.S.," Tables 2 and 3.

21. Stephanie Wasserman, *HIV/AIDS Facts to Consider: 1999* (Washington, D.C.: National Conference of State Legislatures, 1999), 76.

22. Kaiser Family Foundation, "Sex Education in the U.S.," 3.

23. Ibid., 1–2.

24. Centers for Disease Control, "Guidelines for Effective School Health Education to Prevent the Spread of AIDS," *Mortality and Morbidity Weekly Report* 37, s-2 (29 January 1988): 5. Available at http://aepo-xdv-www.epo.cdc.gov/wonder/prevguid/p0000217/p0000217.asp.

25. Ibid., Appendix I.

26. Ibid., 3.

27. Ibid., 2.

28. Karen Hein et al., "Adolescents and HIV: Two Decades of Denial," in *AIDS: Effective Health Communication in the Nineties,* ed. Scott C. Ratzan, (Washington, D.C.: Taylor and Francis, 1993), 222.

29. David L. Kirp, *Learning by Heart: AIDS and School Children in America's Communities* (New Brunswick, N.J.: Rutgers University Press, 1989), 102.

30. Ibid., 225.

31. For background see Josh Barbanel, "Chancellor Has Plan to Distribute Condoms to Students in New York," *New York Times*, 26 September 1990, A1; and Joseph Berger, "5 of Board's 7 for Condoms in the Schools: New York's Chancellor Backed on Distribution," *New York Times*, 27 September 1990, B1.

32. Douglas Crimp and Adam Rolston, *AIDS Demographics* (Seattle: Bay Press, 1990), 62.

33. Rachel Lurie, "Teenagers," in ACT UP/New York Women and AIDS Book Group, *Women, AIDS and Activism* (Boston: South End Press, 1990), 137.

34. Hein et al., "Adolescents and HIV," 222.

35. Ibid., 223.

36. Ibid.

37. Burger, "5 of Board's 7 for Condoms in the Schools," B1.

38. Barbanel, "Chancellor Has Plan to Distribute Condoms," B1.

39. Hein et al., "Adolescents and HIV," 224.

40. United States Conference of Mayors, "Condom Availability in School: Communities Decide," *HIV Capsule Report: Reports of Local Policy Responses to the AIDS/HIV Epidemic*, issue 2, July 1992, 3.

41. Jan Hoffman, "Public Lives: Ex-Chancellor Recalls His Turn on the Hot Seat," *New York Times*, 13 May 1999, B2.

42. Somini Sengupta, "Students Fault Board of Education on AIDS Classes," *New York Times,* 13 March 1997, B3.

43. Edward McCabe, "Our 'Just Say No' School Board," *New York Times,* 30 May 1994, A15.

44. The plans are described in Dave Saltontall, "Crew: Nix Condom Demo," *New York Times*, 10 December 1995, 7; and Jeff Simmons, "Leaders Hit AIDS Teachings," *New York Times*, 19 December 1995, 5.

45. Sengupta, "Students Fault Board of Education," B3.

46. Lynda Richardson, "Condoms in School Said Not to Affect Teen-age Sex Rate," *New York Times,* 30 September 1997, A1.

47. Quoted in Bayer, *Private Acts, Social Consequences,* 220.

48. This prohibition was noted in three different articles in a forum on needle exchange. See A. R. Moss, "Epidemiology and the Politics of Needle Exchange," 1385–87; Roel A. Coutinho, "Needle Exchange, Pragmatism and Moralism," 1387–88; and David Vlahov, "The Role of Epidemiology in Needle Exchange," 1390–92, all in the *American Journal of Public Health* 90, no. 9 (September 2000).

49. Gerald J. Stein, *AIDS Update 2000* (Upper Saddle River, N.J.: Prentice Hall, 2000), 307–08.

50. John W. Fountain, "Protest at Agency Targets Rule on Needle Exchange: Hundreds Rally at HHS for Return of Funding," *Washington Post,* 18 September 1997, A17.

51. John F. Harris, "Policy and Politics by the Numbers," *Washington Post,* 31 December 2000, A1.

52. Chris Collins and Thomas Coates, "Science and Health Policy: Can They Cohabit or Should They Divorce?" *American Journal of Public Health* 90, no. 9 (September 2000): 1389.

53. Stephen Joseph, *Dragon Within the Gates: The Once and Future AIDS Epidemic* (New York: Carroll & Graf, 1982), 114–15.

54. Ibid., 191.

55. Ibid.

56. Ibid., 196.

57. Ibid., 207–08.

58. Ibid., 209.

59. Charles Perrow and Mauro Guillen, *The AIDS Disaster: The Failure of Organizations in New York and the Nation* (New Haven, Conn.: Yale University Press, 1990), 118.

60. Ibid., 120–21.

61. Bruce Lambert, "Drug Group to Offer Free Needles to Combat AIDS in New York City," *New York Times,* January 8, 1988, A1.

62. See Joseph, *Dragon Within the Gates,* 199–200, and Perrow and Guillen, *The AIDS Disaster,* 123, for these differing interpretations.

63. Quoted in Cathy Cohen, *The Boundaries of Blackness: AIDS and the Breakdown of Black Politics* (Chicago: University of Chicago Press, 1999), 206.

64. For a discussion of *New York v. Bordowitz* (25 June 1991) and the necessity defense generally, see Lawrence Gostlin, "Law and Policy," in Jeff Stryker and Mark D. Smith, *Dimensions of HIV Prevention: Needle Exchange* (Menlo Park, Calif.: Henry J. Kaiser Family Foundation, 1993), 53–55.

65. Statement of Gregory Davis speaking as panel member on "The Impact of Syringe Exchange on Communities of Color," Third Annual North American Syringe Exchange Convention, Boston, February 25, 1993.

66. Statement of Ellarwee Garsden speaking as panel member on "The Impact of Syringe Exchange in Communities of Color."

67. Cohen, *Boundaries of Blackness,* 335.

68. For somewhat differing views of the controversy, see Michael Finnegan with Frank Lombardi, "Rudy Urged to Fund Needle Swap," *New York Daily News,* 22 January 1998, 10, and ACT UP, "Mayor's Office Suppressed Report on Expanded Needle Exchange," January 23, 1998, available at www.actupny.org/reports/suppression.html (last accessed 8 October 2000).

69. Raymond Hernandez, "New Law Eases Sale of Needles in an Effort to Curb AIDS," *New York Times*, 6 May 2000, B2; Jaquelyn Swearingen, "Embattled Law Puts Syringes on Shelves," Seattle *Times Union*, 19 December 2000, A1.

70. This certainly is not always the case. Quitting smoking, for example, is an abstinence message that is not steeped in moral considerations. There also are abstinence programs around sexual behavior, for example, that strictly emphasize the practical consequences of extramarital sexual intercourse.

71. Lynda Richardson, "Progress on AIDS Brings Movement for Less Secrecy," *New York Times*, 21 August 1997, A1.

72. Cory SerVaas, "Nettie Mayersohn and her Baby AIDS Bill," *Saturday Evening Post*, January/February 1998, 58.

73. Kevin Sack, "Battle Lines Drawn Over Newborn H.I.V. Disclosure," *New York Times*, 26 June 1994, 23.

74. Joyce Purnick, "When AIDS Testing Collides with Confidentiality," *New York Times*, 18 May 1995, B4; Kevin Sack, "A Debate Over H.I.V. Testing of Newborns Raises a Congressman's Profile," *New York Times*, 17 July 1995, B4.

75. Nat Hentoff, "The Shame of Sheldon Silver," *Village Voice*, 1 August 1995, 18.

76. D. L. Shelton, "Delegates Push Mandatory HIV Testing for Pregnant Women: American Medical Association House of Delegates Vote: Annual Meeting News," *American Medical News*, 26 June 1996, 1.

77. Institute of Medicine, *Reducing the Odds: Preventing Perinatal Transmission of HIV in the United States* (Washington, D.C.: National Academy Press, 1998).

78. Letter from Guthrie S. Burkhead, M.D., M.P.H., to Representative Tom A. Coburn, M.D., 3 February 2000, 2.

79. Nancy A. Wade et al., "Abbreviated Regiments of Zidovudine Prophylaxis and Perinatal Transmission of the Human Immunodeficiency Virus," *New England Journal of Medicine* 339, no. 20 (12 November 1998): 409–14.

80. Letter from Burkhead to Coburn.

81. Ibid.

82. Letter from Representative Tom Coburn to Peter Van Dyke, 9 August 2000, 2.

83. Nettie Mayersohn, "New York Baby AIDS Law Continues to Show Great Success" (press release), 5 September, 2001.

Chapter 5

1. Robert Pear, "Congress Authorizes $875 Million to Fight AIDS in Hard Hit Areas," *New York Times*, 4 August 1990, A1.

2. Letter from the National Organizations Responding to AIDS to all members of U.S. House of Representatives, 31 May 1991.

3. Funders Concerned About AIDS, *Taking Action on AIDS: The Ryan White CARE Act* (New York: Funders Concerned About AIDS, 1995), 6.

4. Mark Donovan, "The Politics of Deservedness: The Ryan White CARE Act and the Social Construction of People with AIDS," in *AIDS: The Politics and Policy of Disease*, ed. Stella Theodoulou (Upper Saddle River, N.J.: Prentice Hall, 1996), 81.

5. Later, to slow the growth of the EMA list, the criteria were changed. An EMA now must have a population of at least 500,000 and have 2,000 AIDS cases reported within the most recent five years.

6. This information comes from a February 21, 1995, letter that the mayor of Boston, Thomas Menino, wrote to Senator Nancy Kassebaum endorsing the 1995 reauthorization.

7. Health Resources and Services Administration, Bureau of Health Resources Development, *Information About the Ryan White Comprehensive AIDS Emergency Act of 1990* (Rockville, Md.: U.S. Department of Health and Human Services, 1990), 9.

8. Robert Buchanan, "HIV Consortia Services Funded by Title II of the Ryan White CARE Act: A Survey of the States," *AIDS and Public Policy Journal* 11, no. 3 (1996): 122.

9. The information in this paragraph is available online from the Department of Health and Human Services. For figures on Title I grant awards, see www.hrsa.dhhs.gov/hab/B/factsheets/title1-2.htm; for information on ADAPs, see www.hrsa.dhhs.hab/B/factsheets/ADAP1.htm.

10. Elinor Burkett, *The Gravest Show on Earth: America in the Age of AIDS* (Boston: Houghton Mifflin, 1995), 151.

11. Ibid., 149.

12. Letter from Nicholas Carballeira to Brian Felt and Denise McWilliams, 19 May 1993, 3.

13. Ibid., 4.

14. The facts recounted here are taken from Gregory Thielemann, Richard Scotch, and Wolfgang Bielefeld, "The Ryan White Act in Dallas," *Policy Studies Journal* 27, no. 4 (1999): 809–25.

15. Cathy Cohen, *The Boundaries of Blackness: AIDS and the Breakdown of Black Politics* (Chicago: University of Chicago Press, 1999), 268.

16. Ibid., 269.

17. Senate Committee on Labor and Human Resources, Ryan White CARE Act Reauthorization: Hearing of the Committee on Labor and Human Resources. 104th Cong., 1st sess. (Washington, D.C.: Government Printing Office, 1995), 66.

18. A full account of Nelson's story appears in chapter 5 of Burkett, *The Gravest Show on Earth*.

19. Letter from Pat Christen to Mario Cooper, 13 June 1995.

20. Letter from Representative Thomas Bliley to members of California congressional delegation, 2 June 2000.

21. Judy Holland, "City Faces Cut in Federal Funding to Fight AIDS," *San Francisco Examiner,* 23 June 2000, A2.

22. Ibid.

23. Terry Beswick, "SFAF Mud Wrestles LA Over AIDS Bucks," *Bay Area Reporter,* 29 June 2000.

24. Carolyn Lochlead, "AIDS Financing Avoids the Ax on Capitol Hill," *San Francisco Chronicle*, 31 July 1995, A1.

25. Government Accounting Office, *HIV/AIDS: Use of Ryan White CARE Act and Other Assistance Grant Funds* (Washington, D.C.: Government Printing Office, 2000), 4. Available at http://frwebgate.access.gpo.gov.

26. Ibid.

27. Ibid.

28. Ibid.

29. Benoit Denizet-Lewis, "Undeterred by Her Critics; Foes Say Head of S.F. AIDS Foundation's High Salary Siphons Money from Services," *San Francisco Chronicle,* 6 September 1999, A17.

30. Cynthia Laird, "Editorial: Another Year, Another Raise," *Bay Area Reporter,* 25 May 2000.

31. Darrin Mortenson, "Federal Funded AIDS Conference Begins Amid Criticism," *Virgin Islands Daily News,* 2 May 2000.

32. Shaun Pennington, "AIDS Conference Makes News for Being in V.I." *Virgin Islands Source,* 31 May 2000.

33. Mortenson, "Federal Funded AIDS Conference."

34. John Marino, "U.S. Corruption Prosecutions Rock Puerto Rico," *Washington Post,* 27 August 2000, A3.

35. Todd Bensman, "FBI Looks at AIDS Clinic's Spending: '98 Audit Targeted Use of U.S. Funds," *Dallas Morning News,* 16 June 2000.

36. ACT UP's San Francisco's actions are colorfully documented on its website (www.actupsf.com). The description here comes from two press releases distributed to AIDⁱ activist e-mail lists. See ACT UP/San Francisco, "ACT UP Urges Congress to Cut AIDS Funding," 29 May 2000, and ACT UP San Francisco, "Censored AIDS Fraud Ad Appears in Roll Call," 22 June 2000.

37. Details of Coburn's positions on the Ryan White CARE Act, as well as pertinent press releases, testimony, and speeches, are available at Coburn's website (www.house.gov/coburn; last accessed 9 October 2000).

Chapter 6

1. See Jon Jeter, "Court Orders AIDS Drugs for Women in South Africa; Efficacy, Distribution Claims by Government Are Rejected," *Washington Post,* 15 December 2001, A24.

2. Justice Edwin Cameron, "The Deafening Silence of AIDS," Jonathan Mann Memorial Lecture, Thirteenth International AIDS Conference, Durban, South Africa, July 10, 2000.

3. The figures and statements regarding Africa are from "USAID CP FY2000: AFR Regional Report," available at www.usaid.gov/pubs/cp2000/afr/afr_over.html (last accessed 2 February 2001).

4. Ibid.

5. These numbers appear in UNAIDS, Joint United Nations Programme on HIV/AIDS, "AIDS Epidemic Update—December 2000," available at www.unaids.org/epidemic_update/report_dec00/index_dec.html (last accessed 5 December 2000).

6. Peter Piot, UNAIDS press release, 7 May 2000.

7. This Publitzer Prize–winning series provides an excellent snapshot of the complex situations created by and creating the AIDS crisis in sub-Saharan Africa. See Mark Schoofs, "AIDS: The Agony of Africa," parts 1–8, *Village Voice,* 9 November 1999–4 January 2000; available at www.villagevoice.com/issues/9952.schoofs.shtml (last accessed 26 January 2001).

8. These figures are from the introduction to Jubilee 2000 Coalition, *Eye of the Needle: The African Debt Report,* November 2000; available at www.jubilee2000uk.org/analysis/reports/needle.htm (last accessed 27 December 2001).

9. Quoted in Joe Lauria, "AIDS Study Cites Dire African Need, $3B Remedy," *Boston Globe,* 29 November 2000, A14.

10. Barton Gellman, "Death Watch: The Global Response to AIDS in Africa; World Shunned Signs of the Coming Plague," *Washington Post,* 5 July 2000, A1.

11. Ibid.

12. Barton Gellman, "An Unequal Calculus of Life and Death," *Washington Post,* 27 December 2000, A1.

13. Gellman, "Death Watch."

14. This story is summarized from Gellman, "An Unequal Calculus of Life and Death."

15. Sabin Russell, "New Crusade to Lower AIDS Drug Costs: Africa's Needs at Odds with Firms' Profit Motive," *San Francisco Chronicle*, 24 May 1999, A1.

16. The idea for the title of this section comes from a reprint of sections of a TAC report covering hearings held by the South African parliament. See Treatment Action Campaign, "If Drug Companies Call Compulsory License Theft, Then We Will Call AIDS Profiteering Murder," reprinted in *Critical Path AIDS Newsletter* no. 34 (summer 2000): 19.

17. U.S. Department of State, "U.S. Government Efforts to Negotiate the Repeal, Termination or Withdrawal of Article 15(C) of the Sought African Medicines and Related Substances Act of 1965," 5 February 1999. Accessed through Consumer Project on Technology website, available at www.cptech.org/ip/health/sa/stdept-feb51999.html (last accessed 5 December 2000).

18. Ibid., 3.

19. Eric Sawyer, written testimony on the role of the U.S. government in combating the global AIDS crisis to hearing of Subcommittee on Criminal Justice, Drug Policy and Human Resources of House Committee on Government Reform, 22 July 1999, 4; available at www.house.gov/reform/cj/hearings/99.7.2/Sawyer.htm (last accessed 15 January 2001).

20. John Siegfried, testimony on behalf of the Pharmaceutical Research and Manufacturers of America before Subcommittee on Criminal Justice, Drug Policy and Human Resources of House Government Reform Committee on U.S. global HIV/AIDS policy, 22 July 1999, 4. Available at www.house.gov/reform/cj/hearings/99.7.22/Siegfried.htm (last accessed 15 January 2001).

21. A more complete record of the back-and-forth correspondence and actions between consumer advocates and the U.S. government appears in James Love's statement in hearings before Congress on the U.S. government's roles in combating AIDS globally. See James Love, "What is the United State's Role in Combating the Global HIV/AIDS Epidemic," statement before Subcommittee on Criminal Justice, Human Resources and Drug Policy of House Committee on Governmental Reform, 22 July 1999; available at www.house/gov/reform/cj/hearings/99.7.22/Love.htm (last accessed 15 January 2001).

22. Vice President Al Gore, letter to Representative James Clyburn, 25 June 1999, 1; available at www.cptech.org/ip/health/sa/vp-feb-25-99.html (last accessed 15 January 2001).

23. David E. Sanger, "Talks and Turmoil: The Overview: President Chides World Trade Body in Stormy Seattle," *New York Times*, 2 December 1999, A1.

24. Office of United States Trade Representative, "The Protection of Intellectual Property and Public Health," press release, 1 December 1999. Available at www.ustr.gov/releases/1999/12/99-97.html (last accessed 15 January 2001).

25. *Congressional Record*, 106th Cong., 2d sess., 27 April 2000, S3039; available at http://thomas.loc.gov/cgi-bin/query (last accessed 27 December 2001).

26. Executive orders have the force of law but do not go through the normal legislative process. Because they are not laws, however, they are limited in the sense that subsequent presidents can overturn the executive orders of their predecessors.

27. Sandra Thurman, testimony before Subcommittee on Criminal Justice, Drug Policy and Human Resources of House Committee on Government Reform, 22 July 1999; available at www.house.gov/reform/cj/hearings/99.7.22/Thurman.htm (last accessed 15 January 2001).

28. Amir Attaran and Jeffrey Sachs, "Defining and Refining International Donor Support for Combating the AIDS Pandemic," *Lancet* 357, no. 9249 (January 6, 2001), 57–61.

29. Raymond W. Copson, "AIDS in Africa," Congressional Research Service issue brief, 20 October 2000, 10–11.

30. Theresa Agovino, "Delegate: AIDS Goal Too Ambitious," Associated Press, 25 June, 2001.

31. The chronology of the pharmaceutical response to the crisis of AIDS in developing countries is described in depth by Barton Gellman, "A Turning Point that Left Millions Behind," *Washington Post,* 28 December 2000, A1.

32. Ibid.

33. Michael Waldholz, "Makers of AIDS Drugs Agree to Slash Prices in the Third World," *Wall Street Journal,* 11 May 2000, A1.

34. "New Public/Private Sector Effort Initiated to Accelerate Access to HIV/AIDS Care and Treatment in Developing Countries," UNAIDS press release, 11 May 2000.

35. "Glaxo Wellcome with Four Other Pharmaceutical Companies Partner with United Nations Agencies in Public/Private Cooperation to Accelerate Access to HIV/AIDS Care in Developing Countries," press release, 11 May 2000.

36. *Medecins Sans Frontieres,* "MSF Statement on New UNAIDS Proposal," 11 May 2000, Paris.

37. Gellman, "A Turning Point."

38. Mark Schoofs and Michael Waldhoz, "Drug Companies, Senegal Agree to Low-Cost HIV Drug Pact," *Wall Street Journal,* 24 October 2000, A1.

39. Kurt Shillinger, "AIDS Plan Offers Africa Hope in Likely Model, Uganda to Receive Cheaper Drugs," *Boston Globe,* 1 December 2000, A1.

40. Alain Guilloux and Suerie Moon, "Hidden Price Taps: Disease-Specific Drug Donations: Costs and Alternatives," Access to Essential Medicines Campaign, *Medicins Sans Frontieres,* October 2000.

41. Gellman, "A Turning Point."

42. Ibid.

43. "US at WHA Colludes with Drug Industry," Health GAP press release, 17 May, 2001. Available at www.healthgap.org (last accessed 20 June 2001).

44. See Charles A. Radin, "Natsios Faces a Firestorm in D.C. Views on Foreign Aid Outrage Advocates," *Boston Globe,* 24 June 2001, A15.

Chapter 7

1. Tina Rosenberg, "Patent Laws Are Malleable. Patients Are Educable. Drug Companies Are Vincible. The World's AIDS Crisis Is Solvable. Look at Brazil," *New York Times Magazine,* 28 January 2001.

2. Ibid.

Index